Matters of the Mind and the Heart

Published by Advantage, Charleston, South Carolina.
Member of Advantage Media Group.

ADVANTAGE is a registered trademark and the Advantage colophon is a trademark of Advantage Media Group, Inc.

Printed in the United States of America.

ISBN: 978-1-59932-063-2
LCCN: 2008921156

Matters of the Mind and the Heart

Meeting the Challenges of Alzheimer Care

Beverly L. Moore

Advantage™

Dedication

This book is dedicated to the many and increasing numbers of families caring for someone with Alzheimer's disease or related memory disorders. You inspired and encouraged me to share your stories.

TABLE OF CONTENTS

Forward

One of my favorite quotes comes from The Little Prince. Author de-Saint-Exupery says, "If you want to build a ship, don't herd people together to collect wood and don't assign them tasks. Rather, teach them to long for the immensity of the sea". Author Beverly Moore has translated that into our new healthcare culture believing that if you want Alzheimer's care to be the best it can be, don't treat family members and home health workers as subordinates and issue them tasks to perform but rather teach them that each has the power to make the life of an Alzheimer family more successful and more fun; help them to learn, on an ongoing basis, to lovingly care for this priceless population who is moving unfaltering toward the final life's chapter

There was a time, not so long ago, when attempts to interact positively with an AD person were scarce and methods on communicating effectively or minimizing behaviors or improving independence were nonexistent. As these new approaches were learned and the benefits to both family members, professionals and patients were noted, appropriate care techniques began to slowly be shared. As a society of professional carepartners, patients, and family members, we must now concentrate on ensuring that the most positive and compassionate living situations are achieved through education and the sharing of best-care practices.

That is the mission of Matters of the Mind – and the Heart. With decades of working in the healthcare field and developing a delightfully outspoken advocacy for Alzheimer patients and carepartners, author Moore brings her pragmatic and compassionate approach to those doing the care and she does so without confusing medical terminology and lofty opinion.

Currently, there is a nationwide cry for culture change in the healthcare system. As Matters of the Mind – and the Heart so nobly demonstrates, this change begins with the inclusion of family members in the decision-making and development of treatment plans; it transcends limited resources and suggests that all families can be taught better ways to care for their loved ones; it creates an atmosphere that fosters learning, responsibility, laughter, and validation. Matters of the Mind – and the Heart underscores the mantra of the national Alzheimer's Association "You are not alone". It is easy for a family member to feel isolated, fearful, frustrated, and fatigued when they lack knowledge of better ways to care. Daily, families watch as this disease erodes tiny bits of a loved one's personality and performance leaving him or her without controls, inhibitions and defenses. Yet this seemingly gloomy scenario can change dramatically when the appropriate responses are learned and positive techniques are implemented.

Training, education, communication, support, and mentoring are the ways that the present culture in healthcare can be changed beginning with the training of one family and continuing until as many families as possible, each year, learn that caring for an Alzheimer person may not be as daunting a task as previously believed and that there is someone with knowledge of the disease and the desire to make the carepartnering experience the best it can be.

Matters of the Mind – and the Heart teaches us all that knowledge really does lead us into a more comfortable, and often glorious, place in our new carepartnering role.

Joanne Koenig Coste, MEd
Author - Learning To Speak Alzheimer's

Acknowledgements

I began writing this book to showcase the many families I've worked with as your coach over the last eight years. There have been some one thousand of you who have taught me the value of family ties. I applaud you and thank you for letting me share your stories of commitment to keep family relationships strong.

For the encouragement to start a business coaching families, I thank Linda George, the creative thinker and executive director of Boston Senior Home Care. Linda was instrumental in presenting and supporting my proposal for the Habilitation Therapy Program to the Executive Office of Elder Affairs of Massachusetts in 1999. This was a new approach to keep elders in their own homes, teaching their care-givers the principles of dementia care and guiding them in learning new approaches to challenges of care.

For the invaluable instruction about behavior I have very grateful thanks for Fred Duhl, MD, my family therapy instructor at the Boston Family Institute in Brookline, Massachusetts. I use the principles of behavior management every day of my life.

Thank you to my husband Curt who gave me space and time to write, who challenged me to finish the book and was willing to go without a few meals now and then.

Thank you to my daughter Becky who, understanding my passion to help families, saw me less often than she or I wanted and made it her business to keep me connected to my five grandchildren.

Thank you to my staff who encouraged me to write, and offered ways to reach people with the good news that Alzheimer's doesn't have to be catastrophic.

Thanks to Judy Paglia, a family caregiver, who graciously permitted me to include her poems. She still misses her dad, her best friend.

Thank you to Sofphronia Scott, the Book Sistah and my writing coach, who taught me the nuts and bolts of writing, publishing and marketing a book. Without her help I'd still be thinking about writing instead of publishing this book.

And a special thanks to God, to Whom I dedicate my work to be honoring His name. He has mightily blessed my work, my family and me.

Still in There

I know he's still in there;
his face is still the same.
The only difference is
he can't remember my name.
But what's in a name?
Should I really care?
For the love we shared
will always be there.

I know he's still in there
behind shining blue eyes;
when he sees a family member
there's the same happy smile,
But he's not the same,
the man he was is gone,
as he waves to the neighbors
and he shuffles 'cross the lawn

-Judy Paglia, caregiver, whose dad had Alzheimer's

Introduction

This is a how-to book: how to care for your family member with memory loss. It explores and explains behaviors, behaviors of people with Alzheimer's disease and those of us who care for them. It is a book about commitment of family to its members. It is a book of love relationships and how people strive to keep them rich in the face of an illness that robs memory.

The lessons contained in this book are told through stories of real people facing new perplexing behaviors, and trying to understand them and to respond to the behavior instead of react. It is not an inclusive book nor is it intended as a scientific or clinical book. It is for people who choose, or find themselves chosen, to care for someone with Alzheimer's or a related memory disorder.

To understand the impact of a memory disorder on life, we need to review some basic concepts of what causes dementia: how damage to certain parts of the brain creates new challenges for the person. But the focus is ultimately on relationships; how to sustain a relationship with that special person you care for. Families I've coached have sometimes found renewed freshness in their love relationship!

There are changes that occur in response to memory loss. They are expressed in new behaviors. All behavior means something: theirs and ours. We must learn an "uncommon common sense," so to speak. I'm here to teach you that new common sense. It will empower you to be more at ease in your role as care partner and to stay in relationship. I heard a saying recently that goes something like this: It isn't the load that wears you down, it's the way you carry it. I will help you carry the load of care partnering differently and more successfully.

My interest in understanding the impact of Alzheimer's disease on a family began in the 1990s when, while developing a mental health program for a home care company, I became aware that the people who were most challenging to serve were those with memory loss and resulting confusion. They didn't remember the person who came to help and, showing good judgment, more often than not, would not allow the helper into the home. This led to my thinking up strategies to get the workers in to give needed care. I subsequently wrote a manual for the workers and developed a spirit of exploration of the world of thinking and behavior.

The Fascinating Brain...

The homecare aides I trained in that program in the nineties learned to work with mentally and/or cognitively impaired elders. People with mental illness, as well as those with dementia, often have memory problems. In class one day I asked the students to think up metaphors to describe their impression of what it must be like to have memory loss.

"It would be like that pesky light bulb that sometimes lights and sometimes doesn't, and you cannot know when it will and when it won't."

"It is like turning on a computer and finding files missing and others mislabeled, and not knowing where to look for information you need."

"I would think people were playing tricks on me, making me look foolish."

We decided to list all the things we could think of that the brain does for us. A large, free-standing white board became filled with words and phrases like plan, initiate, do, think, feel, taste, hear, see, stand, dance, enjoy rhythm, know where we are in space, problem solve, learn, remember, experience emotion, move, swallow, blink, switch subjects, build one concept learned onto a new more complex one, manipulate objects, compensate for loss of function by adaptation, relate to others, think about thinking, use the imagination, know what is real from what is fantasy, fall in love, appreciate the arts, read, write, judge distance and speed (very important in driving and in sports), etc. When we had the board filled to overflowing, I circled then erased one function of the brain after another, asking,

"What would your response be to losing this ability?"

"How would it change your life?"

"How would you act?"

"What would you think was going on?"

"How do you think you would respond to others noticing the change in your ability?"

These are some difficulties the person with early dementia copes with. You can see what confusion, perhaps even panic, it presents for the person. The husband of a woman I coached would sit on the couch in the late afternoon, holding his head in his hands repeating, "I can't think. There is nothing in here anymore." He would proceed to rock back and forth, moaning to himself. He did not want to hear dismissing quips like, "Oh, it's only old age coming on. Don't worry, I have trouble remembering, too. We're just getting 'old timers' disease!" He needed his wife to listen, empathize with him and offer him comfort in her presence, which she learned to do.

When the homecare aides began using these strategies with their clients with memory loss, families unwittingly sabotaged our efforts. Many did not recognize the challenges their family member experienced living each day, and complained about the worker being deceptive.

I soon realized families were generally uninformed about memory loss and the causes of behavioral changes in dementia. They reported having trouble providing care. I began to teach them one at a time about the behaviors of dementia and the reasoning behind our behavior management strategies. They began adopting these approaches, too, reporting that caring was easier and that their interactions with the family member were more satisfying using the new approaches.

When the homecare company closed its doors in 1999, I felt the need to develop a coaching service for families to understand the behaviors of Alzheimer's and related memory disorders. Alzheimer Coaching Services was born January 2000.

Most families rarely seek help to understand new behavior, thinking they ought to know how to care for their family member. So, I began looking for agencies that worked with and could refer these families to us and help fund the service. A valued colleague, Linda George, now executive director of Boston Senior Home Care, was excited about the idea of in-home family education in Alzheimer's care. She encouraged me to write a proposal to the Executive Office of Elder Affairs of Massachusetts to adopt this family educational service as a statewide program. I had never written a formal proposal before, but I boldly requested state funding to help these families. In April of 2000, the proposal was accepted and the Habilitation Therapy Program was launched.

Families who receive the education report now that they not only work differently and more effectively with their family member with memory loss, but that they understand the difference in their interaction. I want to share what families have discovered works to make life understandable and more enjoyable for the person with memory loss and for their care partner, you. The steps of preparation are few: five to be exact. The challenges of care I will explore with you are ten in number. My work is a blessing to me; I hope what this book teaches you will be a blessing to you.

The stories are from my years coaching hundreds of families in metropolitan Boston and surrounding counties. Some families are urban; some live in the country. Some are income poor and some income rich. I've found that no matter what the resources or location, caring for a person you love with memory loss can be emotionally and socially isolating. Coaching is best done on-site in the home.

I have been continually asked by families why they had not been told of these approaches before. Once a relative was given the diagnosis of a memory disorder, families reported they were sent home with little or no information to help them understand the illness or what to expect in daily living. There are classes and seminars on Alzheimer's care, many offered by the Alzheimer's Association, which are valuable; but the particular challenges of a family member's behaviors must be approached one family at a time. Every person with Alzheimer's responds differently.

Together, families and I studied behaviors that were unsafe or that significantly and/or negatively impacted their relationship with their particular family member. Families were encouraged to continue to develop new approaches to changes in behavior based on principles of dementia care as the dementia progressed. I have been touched by their willingness to learn new behavioral approaches in an effort to strengthen family relationships that were strained due to the illness.

Why use stories? We remember stories and relate to them, especially true life stories about people like us. Theories are important, but putting them into action is very personal and the result is often not at all what the theory would suggest. In the moment a new behavior appears, we are not likely to review a theory; we tend to react in our usual way. These approaches and responses are a new way of relating and need to be practiced. Many of these stories will be transferable to your own story.

All of us have a story that needs to be told to benefit others. This is a book about people like you. Read and learn. I am a messenger of good news; you can continue to enjoy a rich relationship with your family member with memory loss.

The Fundamentals of Successful Care Partnering

I don't believe a diagnosis of Alzheimer's or a related memory disorder has to be catastrophic. There are tools to help you go on, and go on well. This is your instruction manual. The requirements for success are a readiness to be a good observer of behavior, a willingness to put your need for credit and recognition for your efforts aside, and the courage to try creative, sometimes seemingly foolish, approaches and interventions.

Understanding of behavior based on new knowledge produces positive feelings of empowerment. "I can make a difference now that I understand" is what I hear again and again. Learning a new way to relate to your family member with memory loss can also ease your grieving for the person that was and help develop and sustain a relationship with who he or she is now.

The following steps are important before we learn how to meet the challenges. Step #1 will give you an understanding of what a marvelous organ the brain is. Step #2 tells you what happens when it is no longer working well. These are essential prerequisites to meeting the several challenges of care. Learning what behavior means is also essential. This is Step #3. You will learn that behavior is not random; it is meaningful. We must learn how to change our behavior. Step #4 teaches you the principles of accommodating to memory loss, and Step #5 prepares you for the impact on family life.

Before we begin, you need to ask yourself these questions. Do I want to learn how relate to my family member with memory loss? Am I willing to take the time to learn how? Will I practice what I have learned and practice bringing to an end reacting out of old habits and expectations? If you answered yes to all the above, proceed toward the steps to good caregiving. Here is Step #1.

Step # 1:
LEARN HOW THE
BRAIN WORKS

What Does the Brain Do, Anyway?

First we need to understand the brain and its functions. Understanding what the healthy brain does helps us understand what happens when it becomes diseased or damaged. All parts of the brain work together to make sense of the world around us and help us work in it effectively. When one part of the brain is injured through trauma or disease, the rest wonderfully accommodates for the loss. However, if the offending condition is progressive, like Alzheimer's type dementia, the brain cannot keep up with the damage caused by the disease. Changes in ability then become more noticeable.

The resilience of the person and their brain is so good that when a diagnosis of Alzheimer's is made, the person usually has had the disease for five or more years. Someone who has had many social connections and continued learning after high school has a more resilient brain; it has a more complex network of nerve pathways to draw on. How wonderful our brain is!

The Healthy Brain

The healthy brain essentially has four functions. It takes in information, processes it, stores it and retrieves it on command.

The brain takes in information. This information may be heard, seen, felt, smelled or tasted. It may be an awareness of another person's intent in relationship to another. It may be a feeling of impending danger or delight.

The brain processes this information to make sense of it, discarding what isn't needed to be able to act on the information. Is this real or not? Is it important to me right now? Is it important to remember? Should I do something now? This allows us to make decisions about how to respond to the information.

That information is then stored so that we don't have to learn it over each time it is presented. And because it is stored, the knowledge can be built on and applied to other things. We learn to ride a bike, balancing our body on two wheels. We transfer this knowledge to balancing on other objects, like skis or a surfboard. We learn to multiply, divide, work with fractions, and use algebra, geometry, trigonometry, calculus and so forth. But we start by mastering addition and subtraction. We can learn how to behave in certain social situations because we've experienced it before and remember the results of our actions.

The brain also allows retrieval of stored information. Over the years we store a lot of information! By middle age, we may have a bit more trouble retrieving things like names or seldom used concepts; but we can retrieve it eventually. For example, I was talking with a client who has been a Red Sox fan since the 1930s. I reminisced with him about the years I enjoyed attending the games in the 1950s with my dad. "Remember, that was when 'what's his name' was in left field," I said. We both tried to recall the name, mentioning other things about the player that might trigger recall. Finally we gave up and went on with the coaching session. A few minutes later, I blurted out, so I wouldn't forget it again, "Ted Williams; he's the left fielder we were thinking of."

We both laughed at this lapse of my memory. He, at eighty-nine, could empathize and enjoy his memory coach's "brain attack."

Step # 2:
LEARN WHAT DEMENTIA IS, HOW THE BRAIN CHANGES

The Unhealthy Brain

All four of these functions—receiving, processing, storing and retrieving—of information are altered in dementia. Some functions are affected more than others depending on what disease or condition is causing the dementia and what part of the brain is damaged. A person affected by Alzheimer's, for instance, will generally have trouble with memory first. A person with frontal-temporal lobe dementia will have memory for some time into the disease but will have socially uncharacteristic behaviors and language deficits. A person who has damage throughout the brain from multi-infarct dementia will have a variety of deficits of language, memory, mood regulation etc.

This is the best reason for a diagnostic workup at a memory clinic or with a physician knowledgeable in cognitive disorders. This may be a geriatrician, a psycho-neurologist, a geriatric psychiatrist or a neurologist who specializes in the cognitive disorders of elders. Knowing what the disorder is helps us to understand how to work with that person.

When affected by dementia, the brain takes in information more slowly, and sometimes not accurately. I liken this to the metaphor of a kaleidoscope. (I often think in pictures, finding it easier to understand a concept, so bear with me if you don't learn this way.) Each primary color in the kaleidoscope represents a bit of information. It is in a certain pattern when we look through the eyepiece, one that is familiar.

In dementia, it is as if someone intermittently rotates the eyepiece, which quickly changes the pattern, making information continually different and new. For the person with dementia, staying in touch with what is happening around them is hard work. The world is a busy place with distractions all about; the kaleidoscope patterns are quickly changing. This further complicates staying oriented and participating in daily life.

Processing information slows as the brain changes due to impaired cognition. Holding onto a piece of information becomes more and more challenging; if it is a progressive memory disorder, the brain soon cannot hold onto information at all. If there is anything distracting during the processing the information may be instantly lost. Information is not forgotten; it never was processed. It is as if it never happened— and for that person, it never did.

Storage of new information is limited, then nonexistent, so retrieval (remembering) is first limited, and then impossible. The part of the brain responsible for retrieval, the hippocampus, has been destroyed, making the person incapable of remembering. So in addition to impaired memory of past learning he or she cannot learn anything new. Quizzing the person in an attempt to help them remember doesn't work. It is very demeaning, pointing out their inability to do so.

The Brain as a Tape Recorder

I've explained memory loss to people this way: The brain is like a tape recorder that contains tapes of everything we have experienced— learned concepts, events, people, places, names, etc. In memory disorders, the tapes are all full with no room to store new experiences. In a progressive dementia like Alzheimer's, memories are erased from the most recently recorded memory to the most remote. Therefore, it is not that the person forgot what you said; it never got recorded. It was never said, as far as he is concerned. This erasure of information is the reason for the repetitious questioning and telling of the same stories over and over. The stories are usually based on the remote past events, which may be distorted and inaccurate. As the disease progresses the person is living in the immediate present. There is no past and no future; just now. You must meet them in the now.

What this means for the person with dementia is this. Paying attention and concentrating become difficult. Distractions become troublesome. Attending to one person's conversation becomes impossible if other people start to talk at the same time; and the person with dementia will surely become lost if those talking switch subjects. Background noises are troublesome and irritating. They are unable to filter out extraneous sights and sounds. Often the person seems to withdraw from social settings, unable to fully express ideas or enter into meaningful, satisfying dialogue.

Language becomes distorted and word finding is harder. Naming objects can be difficult. The person may describe an object instead of naming it. "Can you pass the white sand you put on your food?" Misunderstanding others' intentions is common. Due to slow processing, the person with dementia may respond to something said a minute ago after the conversation is already on another subject. This can make her look more confused than she is. Knowing this, we must accommodate by speaking more slowly and waiting for answers.

Add to this any hearing or vision deficit, and the confusion is compounded. Making sure hearing aids and glasses are provided; it reduces confusion and enhances participation in relationship with others. Not providing these aids causes "excess disability." People who need a cane to walk safely would be at excess disability if we didn't provide them one. The same applies to hearing aids and glasses. Eliminate whatever may further challenge the person to stay in touch with the world about them, and you eliminate excess disability.

Executive (Higher) Function

Multi-tasking is something that normally becomes more challenging as we age. But for the person with brain damage, multi-tasking is downright confusing and frustrating. I knew a colleague who had sustained brain injury to the frontal lobe in a car accident. She described her difficulty in working on a task at her desk. If the phone rang, interrupting her work to answer it, she was unable to pick up the task where she left off, forcing her to go back to the beginning. Even it she left her index finger at the place where she left off, she found she often lost awareness of the goal she was working toward.

Later, working with people with frontal lobe dementia, I found they, too, had difficulty especially in organizing, doing things in the right order (sequencing) and concentrating on a task, especially if multi-faceted. I asked myself, "How can we simplify things so these people experience success with little or no frustration?" (We'll discuss this under Challenge # 2.)

What Part of the Brain Does What?

Let's go through each portion of the brain's cortex (divided into lobes) and learn what each does. As you read, think about activities that damage to that part of the brain would make especially difficult, needing help to ensure success.

The hippocampus, a structure within the temporal lobes (the area that surrounds our ears) is the working memory or relay station of the brain. It takes in information and helps us remember and hold onto information. The temporal lobes process that information, putting together the parts so it makes sense and is useful—or making us aware that it needs to be ignored and discarded. This part of the brain processes language as well, along with the parietal lobes, so we can read, write, understand and use language. The parietal lobes help us identify objects by name and what they are used for. They also enable us to sense heat, cold, pain and touch.

The occipital lobe (back portion of the head) processes information that our eyes see. It tells us how far away something is, how fast something (including ourselves) is traveling, whether a surface is lower or higher than the surface we're on and whether a slope declines or inclines. It shows us how to get from one place to another. This ability to find our way around is called cognitive mapping: the ability to hold onto a map in our head. Without this mapping we would get lost, not knowing whether to go right or left to get home (or even perhaps to find the bathroom!). A person with damage in this lobe may have a hard time sensing where they are in space, and sit in thin air a foot away from the chair next to them.

The frontal lobe is responsible for the higher "executive" functions of thinking; initiating, planning, organizing, sequencing, making social decisions, regulating mood, and responding to the environment responsibly and appropriately. These are important functions to help us deal with our daily living activities. The cerebellum, the pons and the medulla are responsible for balance, breathing, body temperature regulation, heartbeat, swallowing, digestion and other basic life sustaining functions. These latter parts are usually, if at all, affected late in a progressive dementia.

What Does the Word Dementia Mean, Anyway?

Let's talk a bit about the term dementia. I hear people say, "The doctor said he doesn't have Alzheimer's disease; he has dementia." The next question should be, "What is causing the dementia?"

Dementia is simply a descriptive term that means persistent cognitive decline—signs (what others notice) and symptoms (what the individual reports) that indicate he isn't able to do things well or easily. Signs are those changes that family and friends may notice; that the individual has lost interest in doing things he had previously found pleasurable. They may also note confusion (a mixed up order of things or getting lost in a task), trouble solving everyday problems (inability to make a simple meal or get dressed), impaired judgment and logic (continuing to drive after several accidents or crossing a busy street without looking), memory loss, an inability to initiate meaningful activity or organize and complete tasks, speech problems, and difficulty doing things that have previously been easy for them.

Symptoms are those changes the person notices. She may say, "I just don't quite feel myself. I'm having more difficulty doing things. It is hard to cook, and I'm getting confused making change at the grocery store." Generally others notice changes before the person with dementia does. Perhaps it happens so gradually that the person isn't even aware she is changing.

What Causes Dementia?

Dementia can be caused by any condition—a physical condition like a disease or an environmental situation like working with toxins. Any disease that deprives the brain of oxygen, prevents adequate nutrition or fails to free the body of toxins can cause brain changes. Some diseases that may cause signs of dementia are heart and lung disease preventing adequate oxygen perfusion, intestinal disorders that prevent absorption of nutrients, alcoholism, kidney disease and liver disease (the liver is the filter for the body to get rid of toxins). Diseases like Parkinson's, multiple sclerosis, Huntington's, AIDS, diabetes, hypothyroidism (inadequate thyroid function) and, the most well known, Alzheimer's disease, can or do cause dementia. Environmental causes for dementia may include a long work history handling and inhaling toxins, for example working with epoxy in the boat building business. Chronic drug or alcohol abuse and smoke inhalation can also cause dementia. The dementia caused by alcohol abuse is called Korsakov's disease.

Unless caused by some sudden trauma to the head, such as stroke or an accident, dementia is recognized slowly over time. Undiagnosed concussions from sports injuries or motor vehicle accidents can predispose a person to dementia. Repeated trauma to the brain kills brain cells from inflammatory processes.

Families often attribute changes in thinking to lack of sleep, stress, depression, irregular or burdensome work schedules, or changes in lifestyle (children leaving home, death of a spouse, retirement, a move or a reduction in financial resources). Changes may be ignored or minimized for some time. A crisis brings awareness.

Pause for thought

What risks in your life could predispose you to dementia? Can you reverse the risks by lifestyle changes?

_____

_____

_____

_____

Is a Diagnosis Important?

The importance of a definitive diagnosis cannot be overstated. Cognitive changes, as we've discussed, have so many causes that everything that could be the source of trouble must be ruled out before an accurate diagnosis can be made. There are some conditions that cause signs and symptoms of dementia that can be treated effectively and sometimes reversed.

A definitive diagnosis of Alzheimer's disease is made by exclusion. Every condition that could contribute to the cognitive changes noticed is eliminated to arrive at a diagnosis of Alzheimer's. This diagnosis of probable Alzheimer's is found to be 85-95 percent accurate; the only absolute diagnosis is made on examination of brain tissue at autopsy. Obviously no one wants a brain biopsy until then!

Donating your brain to research is a great contribution to furthering knowledge of Alzheimer's disease and related disorders. Much of what we have learned about what happens to the brain has been from the study of donated brains. The Nun Study taught scientists much from the study of nun's lives, their behavior and how it related to the damage seen on autopsy. These nuns were all from the same convent. Some had signs of dementia while others were clearly cognitively sound. You can find the results of this study on the Internet under Alzheimer's.

The diagnostic evaluation can be done by a geriatrician, a neurologist, a neuropsychologist or a primary care doctor skilled in dementia. There are memory clinics in many hospitals across the country and the world that provide a diagnostic workup. These can be found through the Alzheimer's Association website. The national association's website is www.alz.org.

A correct diagnosis is important for planning treatment, including preventive measures. A person with vascular dementia, for instance, will want to keep his blood pressure under control and continue to take any medications that improve heart function to avoid further small strokes or a major one. Some medications for one kind of dementia are contraindicated, maybe even potentially lethal, in other dementias like Pick's disease and Lewy body disease.

Someone with poor judgment from dementia will need her medication and diet to be carefully monitored for ultimate protection from further brain damage. A person with mood regulation problems caused by frontal lobe dementia will need a calm environment. Each person with dementia has deficits peculiar to him or her, so each person needs to have an individualized treatment and care partnering plan. Carepartnering is a coined phrase that suggests that we care for a person by partnering with them, whereas caregiving suggests that we do for them instead of engaging them in their own care. We will discuss carepartnering plans later when we look at the challenges of dementia.

Let's review what is different in dementia thinking.

- Processing information from the surroundings may be distorted and may misrepresent what is being said in conversation.

- Retaining or holding onto a piece of information is hard.

- Concentrating is possible only if one simple activity (sometimes one step of an activity) is presented calmly.

- Filtering out background noises and attending to something is difficult.

- Storing (memory) and retrieving (remembering) information is slower. The person may fail to recognize familiar people, have trouble doing familiar tasks or fail to recognize what an object is or what its use is.

• Organizing tasks that must be done in the right order of logical sequence is harder. (This is frontal lobe executive function.)

• Awareness of surroundings lessens in a progressive cognitive disorder.

• Awareness of the passage of time is affected. The person may lose contact with the time, day and season. This results in much confusion.

• Interest in things that previously had brought pleasure lessens. The person may give up reading, knitting, golf, etc.

• Initiating a task, an activity or conversation is lessened to avoid failure and/or due to brain changes.

Pause for thought

Before going on, think of 3-5 ways you feel would help the person you care about stay in touch with what is going on around them.

_____

_____

_____

_____

_____

Step # 3:
LEARN ABOUT BEHAVIOR AND ITS MEANING

Behavior Means...

It is essential for us to learn about behavior and its meaning. Behavior is how we express our wants, our needs and our feelings. We need to be aware of our own behaviors and try to understand the behaviors of others. As dementia care partners, you can change your knee jerk reaction to behaviors you find perplexing, unpleasant or perhaps annoying, and learn to respond thoughtfully in a helpful way. This is the reason for Step #3.

The goal in understanding dementia behavior is to respond instead of reacting to daily situations. This enables you to create opportunities for successful living and support for your relationship with that person. This takes practice. The longer your history together, the more practice is needed to change; but your behavior can and must change in order for you to find enjoyment in caring. The person with dementia cannot alter his behavior due to brain changes; you must take the responsibility to change your behavior.

Pause for thought

What behaviors of others are most troublesome to you? What triggers you to react in ways that may not be helpful as a care partner?

_____

_____

_____

_____

Principles are guides to action. Understanding behavior can help overcome our reacting to situations that are toxic to us and help us to respond in a more productive way. We encounter all kinds of situations in life, outside carepartnering, that challenge us. If a car cuts you off on the highway going eighty-five mph, what is your immediate reaction? If you went by that first reaction, what would be the end result? You might want to chase the car and let the driver know what you think about his driving. Is this a safe way to react? You might want to blow your horn loudly at him. Or, you might just shrug and say, "Wow, that was close! I hope he gets where he's going in such a hurry."

Why did you do what you did? Was your action based on past experience? We change our behavior when we learn that what we did do doesn't work effectively anymore.

Pause for thought

Think of reactionary (knee-jerk) behavior of yours you'd like to change to a more effective one.

_____

_____

_____

_____

_____

Guidelines to Understanding Behavior: Ours and Others'

Let's look at some principles of behavior: what it is, why we do what we do and how to change our behavior and others'.

- Behavior always means something; it is goal-directed, designed to make something happen. This goal can be realized consciously or unconsciously. For example: Why do you park at that particular end of the store's parking lot?

Why do you prefer to take the scenic route even though it takes longer? What is the goal? Are the things you usually buy at that end of the store? Does the scenic route relax you before you get to your destination? Are these goals conscious, or do you just do them without thinking about it?

- Behavior is context defined; we behave differently in different places We don't share thoughts and feelings the same way with a stranger like we do with our dearest friend, nor do we behave in a grocery store the same as we might at a party or in a house of worship.

- Behavior is learned; it is how we take charge of our life. If we learn that being brash and demanding gets us what we want, we will no doubt continue to be demanding. If we find that being polite and modest is instrumental in getting our needs met, we will no doubt continue this behavior.

- Behavior can change. When a behavior doesn't produce what we want anymore, we will behave differently. People who cut in line usually get to be first. Others are annoyed but may not say anything. But if those people actually spoke up, do you think the pushy person might pause before cutting in line next time? You bet!

- To change a person's behavior, we must change the way we respond to the behavior. Then the behavior will change—maybe not exactly the way we would like, but it changes.

I worked with single mothers for several years as an outreach therapist. Once the referral was nineteen-year-old mother who had been reported by the neighbors for the daily yelling coming from her house. This young mother's four-year-old would demand her attention when she came home from pre-school each day. She would hang on her mother's dress, whining and crying for attention. This annoyed the mother, who wanted to watch her favorite soap opera that began at three. Throughout the program there was a battle: the mother telling the child to leave her alone, and the child, screaming to be heard. I learned that the child usually got off the bus at two forty-five, fifteen minutes before the TV show began. I suggested to the mother that she spend fifteen minutes listening to her child's day, asking her for pictures she'd drawn, and I suggested they have a snack together. What did the child want: closeness with her mother, and attention. When the mother gave her these things before the child had to "act" to get it, she was child satisfied and ready to play elsewhere by three. The yelling ceased and each person got what she wanted.

Here, I'd like to acknowledge a great teacher who first taught me these principles when I was a family therapist trainee. Fred Duhl, M.D., is a psychiatrist and a musician as well as a magician (really) who taught family therapy using metaphor and behavior management strategies. I've used the principles he taught me successfully in mental health nursing, in family work, in coaching and in my personal life. Thank you again, Fred!

Behaviors of People with Memory Loss

The behavior of cognitively impaired persons is the end result of a combination of two factors. First, they respond out of the coping style that brought success in getting their needs met in the past. Second, they will do things because part of the brain is not giving them the right information or allowing them to do something.

Their behavior is also very dependent on what is going on around them. If the environment feels threatening, there will be a reaction to that. And, a confused person generally and frequently reacts, rather than responding by asking for clarification!

Many if not most people eventually become unaware of their cognitive deficits after the early stage of the disease or condition causing dementia. So, persons with dementia do something to make sense of out their new world. They may confabulate (make up a story to explain why they did something or thought something to be true), or deny they did something, often with no memory of having done it. They are not lying or trying to be manipulative. They may withdraw from engaging with other people. They may become angry when confronted about their behavior, argue with your perception of the situation at hand, dissolve in tears or maybe simply leave the place that is causing them confusion. Their behavior is often perplexing because it doesn't seem to make sense. Think of it this way: the behavior is a way to stay in charge of their world.

Most behaviors of those with dementia are simply the person's way of responding to the now new confusing world they find themselves in. Familiar places and people may become less familiar; unfamiliar things are often frightening, perhaps at times terrifying. She becomes lost in conversation if we don't accommodate the changes in her thinking. Feeling left out, she may act on that feeling without being able to explain what she is feeling.

The overriding emotion of people with dementia is fear: fear of the unknown, fear of failing or being caught in an error, fear of looking foolish, fear of feeling lost, or fear of being abandoned. He may sense that he is becoming a burden to you. Fear may result in his reluctance to engage in activity alone or with others, even people he knows well. This reticence may be demonstrated passively by withdrawing, or actively by aggressive behaviors. Aggression is often the expression of fear.

Just a word about late afternoon—this is often a hard time for people with dementia. The phenomenon of becoming more confused or agitated is called "sundowning." Some experts think this is caused by light changes in the late afternoon, perhaps when shadows make the environment look different. This can evoke a visual hallucination (a false apparition) that is frightening. I also think it may be that the person is so tired staying in touch with what is happening that she is more emotionally vulnerable. At this time, just about anything frustrating to her can trigger a negative behavior. This sundowning phenomenon is like a toddler's meltdown when she becomes tired at the end of the day. It is the outcome of a busy or difficult day.

Initiative wanes as dementia progresses; perhaps partly so that the affected person can defend themselves against failure, and partly because of damage to the brain. He cannot think up something to do or organize himself to begin. This means that he needs us to structure his day more as the disease progresses. We must learn to accommodate him; he cannot accommodate us.

Step # 4:
LEARN WAYS TO ACCOMMODATE A PERSON WITH MEMORY LOSS

Learn Uncommon Common Sense

There are ways you can help your carepartner (care recipient) stay in touch with what is going on around them and participate more fully in everyday life. Some seem like common sense, but remember that this person is someone you care about and have related to perhaps for years. Relating is emotion-charged for you. It takes effort to relate in a different way, remembering that she has changed. You need to learn to care for her as she is now, letting go of who she was.

Couples who have been together for many years have a major challenge learning new ways because they have related in a particular way for decades. If you've been with your partner for years, you know what I'm talking about. She gets a certain look on her face; you stop talking. You behave a certain way; he knows your feelings are hurt. I liken it to a dance (yes, another metaphor): when dementia changes one partner's thinking, the dance changes, steps are lost and confusion results.

Adult children can often adjust easier to relating in a new way, perhaps because they have been separated by distance from their parents or are less emotionally involved as life gets busier and contact less frequent. But either way, whether you are in an intimate relationship or not, you can learn a new way.

As a coach, I find that once care partners understand the meaning of the changes in ability—that the person they are caring for cannot do certain tasks anymore because the brain won't allow them to—and become interested in connecting to the person they care for, they are motivated to try new ways. When they experience better responses from their partner, they continue to practice, especially when they note a happier, less frustrated partner. Some become experts!

So here are some hints to help you help him or her stay connected and capable of engaging in life with you.

Visual Cues

A visual cue is something a person will respond to appropriately because he sees it. We all use visual cues to remind us of things we want to remember. We might put out our morning medications on the counter to remember to take them, or put our keys in a certain place so we don't have to look for them when we leave in the morning for work. My keys, garage door opener, glasses and phone are in a bright purple basket right next to my saucer with my morning vitamins.

Where do you put your keys, glasses, wallet, pills?

Visual cues work because:

- Visual cues tap memory of over-learned behaviors (those we do without thinking because we've done them often for so long).

- A visual cue "jump starts" the brain to remember what to do when presented with that cue. Putting a broom into her hand and asking her to sweep the kitchen, is more successful than simply asking her to sweep the kitchen, especially if the broom is out of view.

• Keeping something that is unsafe out of view can be helpful in maintaining safety because out of sight often means out of mind. This may include knives, guns, power tools, toxic solutions, car keys and the automobile.

• Mirroring is a visual cue. For example, a person may have trouble using eating utensils. If we sit across from him, using the utensils correctly, it can facilitate his continuing to eat with a fork, knife and spoon. It also helps to simplify the setting, putting out only what is needed. That also helps his concentration.

Tips for creating a successful experience:

• Stay focused, with no distractions.

• Turn off competing noises; maintain calm quiet.

• Do one thing at a time, maybe one step at a time.

• Avoid chatty talk when working at a task

• Avoid introducing novelty into a task; she cannot develop skill in new ways of doing things.

• Do the activity with them. A person with dementia cannot attend to a task long without guidance.

Mood Is Contagious

We are all affected by others' moods; if we look at a person with a smile and a hello, they more often than not return the smile. The person with dementia is very sensitive to mood and may lack the ability to perceive what the mood of another person is to respond to it effectively. If you are deep in thought, head down with a furrowed brow, for example, he may ask you, "Are you angry with me?"

Tips for creating a positive mood:

- Calmness in the care partner creates a calmer mood in the person with dementia, so stay calm.

- Conversely, negative mood can be evoked by anything or anyone that creates anxiety for the person with dementia.

- Avoid argument; you will lose. A person with slow processing cannot sustain an argument, so she will repeat something over and over until she wears you down. A few moments later she will have no memory of the argument but you suffer the emotional aftermath (usually guilt) of having sustained (or started) the argument.

- Satisfy the immediate emotional need; this may be a need for comforting, acknowledgement of his value, or clarification of something confusing or frightening.

Determining what the immediate emotional need is can be tricky. You need to be familiar with the person, know whether he needs affirmation, recognition, a feeling of being loved, being in control, comfort, or a need for guidance. Perhaps the person wants to be left alone, enjoying quiet time! If you know the person you are caring for, you will encounter the same needs he had when well. If you don't know him well, those that do can help you understand his needs.

Tips for creating a positive response:

- Create a pleasant atmosphere. She will remember the pleasant feeling of it, and sometimes being in a place she doesn't want to be can be eased by supplying something enjoyable to do.

- Make him feel good when with you. He may not know who you are, but he will know how good it feels to be with you.

- Create fun. She may not remember an event but she'll be left with a positive feeling. She may even remember the event because it was so enjoyable!

Use Humor

Watch how you use humor. Sometimes it is misunderstood and can cause confusion or an unwanted response, so monitor the response.

I like to try a joke with someone to assess their level of awareness and to see if they still understand humor and can respond to it appropriately. I tell this lame joke: Question: What did the man do when his cat was run over by a steamroller? Answer: He did nothing; he just stood there with a long puss.

One gentleman I saw in his home appeared to be out of touch with his surroundings. He looked vacant and lost, sitting in a dark corner of the room with seemingly no awareness. I was there speaking with his wife, and I turned to him and said, "I have a silly joke. I'll tell it to you. Maybe you'll like it." When I told him the joke, he burst into laughter and said, "That joke is pathetic!" He was not so out of touch after all! He subsequently joined us at the dining room table and participated in the conversation some. We just needed to make the effort to connect first.

On the other hand, I had been joking for some time with a nursing home resident during my visits. We both bantered and used soft sarcasm at times. One day, she was very grouchy, resisting the resident aide's effort to guide her to the dining table. I stopped and said laughingly, "Whoa, are you in a grouchy mood today! Don't take it out on Tom." She responded with a snap, "Don't talk to me that way. You're nobody." Naturally I was taken aback, but then I realized I had overstepped our relationship. Bantering was only good when she was in the mood. I sought her out after she was settled, and apologized. She said she'd think about accepting my apology!

Use "Fiblets"

Fiblets are little untruths that benefit the person with dementia. Many carepartners have difficulty using this strategy, arguing that they've always been honest and trustworthy with the person and cannot lie. Fiblets, however, are always to benefit the person with dementia; they are not used to tell untruths for any other reason.

- Get into his present reality and stay there (the immediate present is all there is for someone with severe memory loss).

- Fiblets can help satisfy an emotional need. For example, if a woman believes her deceased mother is still alive and that she has to wait for her, your telling her that her mother called and said she'd meet the two of you later in the day can relieve her worry. Counting on memory loss, you've satisfied her need to include her mother and also avoided argument about whether her mother is alive or deceased!

We'll talk more about this when we look at anecdotes that demonstrate the usefulness of fiblets to meet some of the challenges of care.

Avoid Long Explanations

Logic and reason won't be processed by someone with dementia and will only cause frustration. Logic is too complex to grasp, and reasoning further complicates conversation. Frustration caused by lengthy explanation is sometimes the reason for agitation which can lead to aggressiveness. He is simply getting rid of the frustrating element...you!

Tips to help them feel valued:

- Inform and orient but do not correct ideas or test memory by quizzing. If you say, "It's time for bed," and she says, "I just awoke; I want to eat breakfast. I want cereal," it is probably wise to make a breakfast snack for her and bring up bedtime a little later. Maybe get into your pajamas as a visual cue. Trying to convince her it is nighttime is useless.

- All people need to feel valued; avoid pointing out errors in their reasoning or logic.

- If you find yourself explaining something, remember to "zip your lip." Explanation is a wasted effort that will only lead to frustration for both of you. Simply state a request. "It is time to go." Don't say why you need to go; simply that you're going.

- If you see a confused look on his face as you are talking, you are talking too much; he is lost.

Give Choices Whenever Safely Possible

All people need to sense meaning and purpose to continue to want to participate in life.

- Give no more than two choices, either of which is okay with you.

  —"Do you want to eat now or wash up first?"

  —"Do you want eggs or cereal for breakfast?"

  Even if he makes no choice at all, leaving it up to you, that is still a choice! He's chosen not to choose.

- If memory loss is immediate, mention the choice you want her to make last. Most times that is what she will "remember" and will choose that. So, if you only have eggs and none of her favorite cereal, you might say, "I'd like eggs and toast this morning. Instead of cereal, will you join me? I'm having eggs and toast." More often than not, the invitation to join you will bring out a yes.

Learn New Responses

This attitude helps you look at "problem behaviors" in a different light—one of curiosity about what the behavior means. Behavior has always been an interest of mine, which has helped me in that few behaviors are really annoying to me; and if they are, I respond differently from what is expected.

For example, I cannot tolerate a screaming child. One of my grandsons was very emotionally labile when he was a toddler (high maintenance is how we described him). If something didn't go his way, he would give the most bloodcurdling scream to protest. One day, exasperated with his behavior, I simply said to him, "That is a pathetic scream. Even I can do better than that." And I proceeded to scream in his face. He looked at me, dumbfounded, then screamed back even louder. I continued, "I can yell louder than you; you're little and I'm big." And I did. We got into a screaming contest and both ended up hoarse; then, looking at each other's contorted face, we cracked up laughing, he rolling on the floor and me rocking next to him, holding onto my sides.

When he was just a bit older and verbal, he learned that he could change his behavior. If he felt he was "losing it," he would say, "I am going upstairs until my feelings feel better." If I called up, asking if he was ready to join the family again, he might call back, "No, my feelings are not feeling well enough yet."

Think of their behavior this way:

- Behavior is an expression of emotional or physical need. Satisfy the immediate emotional need. Crying, for example is an expression of need for attention, soothing or perhaps empathy. Crying may be the only way the confused person is able to express frustration.

- Look beyond the behavior to what is being expressed in feeling.

For example: 'Home' is a place of emotional safety. We no doubt feel most at ease in our homes. When someone with memory loss says he wants to go home, he's saying he is feeling emotionally or physically unsafe. Create a safe environment for him. Reassuring him that he is safe with you often works to calm an anxious person.

A care partner related this observation to me: she notices that her husband can no longer initiate activities that are meaningful to him. He relies on her to guide him throughout the day. When she dresses in clothing that points out she is going out that day (a visual cue learned long ago), he becomes huffy and short with her. His behavior hurts her (she thinks she deserves a day out—and she does), but she knows that this behavior is expressing his uneasiness in structuring his day by himself. She has since arranged to have someone be there when she gets dressed, and stay to do things with him while she is gone.

Use Memory Loss to Defuse the Situation

Her memory loss can work for you as carepartner. Assess how short her memory is and use that knowledge to recreate calm in the midst of a storm!

- If the present situation is toxic or frustrating because an immediate need isn't being met, redirect him to something that is pleasant; and often memory of the previous frustrating situation will disappear.

- Sometimes your behavior will appear unkind to the untrained eye. For example, while you are ending a visit with a person with immediate memory loss who gets fretful when you leave, telling a fiblet can be a very kind act. You can tell her that you are simply stepping out of the room for a moment to talk with someone when actually you are leaving. You know that as soon as you are out of sight (you are the visual cue), you were never there! This way you leave her in a positive mood. Obviously this cannot be used if short term memory is still intact. That would then be rightfully viewed as unkind. It can be hard for you to leave her without a hug or kiss, but giving a hug would be a cue that you were leaving, defeating the goal of your fiblet, which is to leave her in a positive frame of mind.

Tips to appeal to sexuality in dementia care:

People continue to be sexual beings throughout life. We do not cease to be men or women when our cognition changes.

- Create a sense of worth and affirm his masculinity or her femininity by our actions. Continue your usual expressions of affection.

- Affirm her sexuality with hugs, a kiss or hand holding. This says she is still attractive to you.

- Some behaviors that appear sexual may have another meaning. For example, if a man tugs at his pants' zipper, or wiggles or rubs his genitals, he may simply need the toilet and not know how to tell you. Do not reprimand; take him to the bathroom! You may add, "Is this what you need?" The visual cue of the room may be all he needs to complete toileting.

I heard of one gentleman in a nursing home who allegedly reached for staff members' breasts. Staff would reprimand him (not a good response) and lead him to a chair, often under severe resistance. He would become angry and combative at these times. Administration called in a consultant, a woman, who approached the gentleman to assess his behavior. As he reached out, she decided to wait to see what his intentions were. He reached up and touched her name badge on her left breast, picked it up and read her name. "So your name is

Barbara." He then put down his hand to shake hers and invited her to walk the hall with him.

It is entirely possible that someone's behavior has been wrongly viewed as sexual when it is in reality an attempt to connect socially.

I also heard about a gentleman who resided in the memory unit in a nursing home. He was typically easygoing, so when an aide noticed him restless, she asked him, "Do you need the bathroom?" He replied, "Yes, I do. Can you take me there?" The aide led him to the bathroom and started to help him unzip his trousers, a task he often had difficulty with. She was shocked when he hit her. Staff came to defuse the situation, asking him if he knew why he hit her. His answer was, "I just wanted to wash my hands; what was she doing unzipping my pants? I was scared."

It would have been better (and safer) if she had asked, "Do you need help?" He would then have indicated by his actions what his trip to the bathroom was for. The lesson is to ask questions that can be answered yes or no, and to ask them throughout a task. This gives you clear direction and gives him choices. Never assume you know; ask.

Pause for thought

What behaviors of your family member with memory loss are perplexing to you? What behavior would you like to understand and work on a new approach to?

_____

_____

_____

_____

Step # 5:
LEARN HOW ALZHEIMER'S AFFECTS FAMILY LIFE

Be Ready for Change—Don't Resist It

Family relationships shift when members become aware of changes in ability and behavior that signals possible dementia. The signs of change in cognition are subtle and are easily "explained" away by family members. Some assume, in error, that it is normal aging. Memory loss and confusion are never normal aging.

Families may reason that these changes in ability or behavior are due to recent changes in the person's life like retirement, a newly diagnosed condition or illness, loss of a job, death of a spouse or perhaps the stress of moving to a new home. But minimizing or denying memory loss is counter-productive.

Family members may be in conflict over how serious the changes are. Some will be proactive and seek diagnosis and treatment; others will avoid being involved, perhaps saying, "I saw her yesterday and she looked fine to me." These differences, if preventing a course of action that is needed for safety and health, can be addressed by a dementia coach, a counselor, or mediation service.

Impact of Early Stage Signs and Symptoms on Family Life

There may be lapses of memory or confusion about appointments. The person may get lost driving to a familiar place. I heard of one gentleman who drove himself to the doctor's office (he had several doctors) on the wrong day at the wrong time and to the wrong doctor. This error was repeated several times before the family sought help to understand this behavior and learn how to help him with his confusion.

Another client left her home to visit her brother who lived five miles away, only to arrive five hours later in a town two hundred miles northwest. While filling up with gas, she asked how to get back to where she lived. She was told "southeast." She drove in the suggested direction only to arrive in a major city ninety-five miles south of her hometown. Her family, wanting her to continue driving, excused that trip as a fluke and insisted she was capable of continuing to drive. The fact that her car's side mirrors were replaced time and time again indicated that she had a distorted sense of space and distance. She had no memory of these events. This family's denial could eventually have caused her death or another person's.

It is never helpful to ignore the signs of dementia. You can see that some areas of her cognition were still intact. She brought money, stopped for gas at the appropriate time and ate in restaurants along the way, but had no sense of where she was in time and space.

Poor logic or judgment may be noticed. Often this change is seen before memory loss. He may do things that seem risky or unsafe yet seem unaware that it was unsafe. We have all left the coffee maker on and gone to work only to come home to a strong coffee smell. (At least I have done this; how about you?) If this happens over and over and he does not sense it is anything to be concerned about, it may indicate a change in judgment.

Often lack of logic concerning money is noticed. She may withdraw money from the ATM daily, forgetting she had done so yesterday, and then argue with the bank teller that he is stealing her money when she sees the balance.

Changes in language can be an early sign. The person may get lost in conversation. He may have difficulty following the gist of conversation or be unable to adapt when the subject changes. This behavior is often explained away by families, who blame it on hearing loss, disinterest, selfishness or rudeness—or simply being contrary. If any of these had historically been personality traits, it is easier for family to fail to notice it as a deficit in his thinking.

We usually continue to use the coping style that has served us best until it doesn't work anymore. And, most traits and coping styles are more pronounced in dementia, not changed. You and I might realize that an old way of relating is not working anymore, and try to change to something different. The person with memory loss doesn't recall the situation that would have taught her that, and she continues to behave in the same ineffectual way.

Any change may create alarm for the family that "something is wrong," or the family may erroneously assume it is age-related memory changes. Again, memory loss is never normal aging. There is forgetfulness, yes, but memory loss, a definite no. It always has a cause (refer back to the section on causes of dementia).

I've heard the difference between memory lapse and memory loss explained this way. A person goes shopping at the mall. Several hours later she doesn't remember where she parked her car. She retraces her shopping venture in her mind and remembers she came in the south entrance. She leaves by that way and finds her car. That is memory lapse, or forgetfulness. Another person goes shopping and parks her car. After a few hours of shopping, she decides to go home. She doesn't remember she came in a car, so she hails a cab and goes home to discover that "someone has taken her car." That is the difference; the memory of the trip to the mall is lost, not just hard to retrieve.

The person with dementia may become defensive, especially when embarrassed or criticized. Often he is quite unaware of the impact their cognitive decline has on everyday living. He may even say, "I have Alzheimer's," and still be totally unaware of his behavior change.

Others are very aware of their disease, but still unaware of their behavior changes. Recently a woman greeted me at the door, noting the sign Alzheimer Coach on my car bumper. "I guess I'm your patient. I have Alzheimer's." In discussion with her and her husband of sixty-six years, she kept asking him, "Did I do that? I don't remember," when he related stories of her strange new behaviors. "The kids were here last night? Where was I?" She wasn't defensive, just puzzled. She is an easy person to work with for her family. Most people with dementia become defensive when their behavior changes are discussed. They have no memory of the behavior and will argue they didn't do that!

Frustration with trying to stay in touch with what is happening around them may cause a person to withdraw or to lash out. These different reactions, again, depend on coping style. Some will stay in bed if they awaken and have no idea how to start their day.

People with dementia may become confused or bewildered about what is happening to them. The people I've met said they thought they were going crazy or were stupid. Neither, of course, is the case. They need reassurance that these things are not true. It is important to allow conversation about how they feel about what is happening to them.

I've spoken with many people in the early stages (and later stages as well) who complain that no one will talk with them about their condition and its impact. "Suddenly I'm invisible. People talk about me in front of me but not to me." I tell them, "I'm still here!"

If a person expresses a wish to tell you what it is like for them, listen! Do not attribute it to aging or say something like, "I forget things, too." This is not what they need; they need to be heard. Consider how you might feel if your thinking changed.

There are early stage support groups where people can talk about how it feels to be in the world with dementia. You can find them on the Alzheimer's Association website, www.alz.org.

Relationships Shift

As relationship roles shift, especially with couples in long-term relationships, feelings will emerge that must be expressed to avoid conflict and hurt. For example, the partner who took charge of maintaining the home, the social calendar, travel arrangements, car maintenance and repairs and investments or other financial decisions may feel left out or "dismissed" if the spouse assumes that role, especially prematurely. It may have been a coveted role for the person with the diagnosis, giving him status. The partner who takes over the role may be happy to do so, or find confidence in doing it and fail to acknowledge the loss for the diagnosed partner. Old issues of who is in control may raise their ugly heads again. If this creates persistent conflict and can't be talked about, the care partner should seek professional help from a coach or counselor who understands the grief everyone experiences in dementia, the one with the diagnosis and those who care about him.

The Challenge of the Independent Minded Person

The response the affected person has to dementia is, as we've said previously, twofold: the parts of the brain damaged, and the person's coping style and personality traits. A person who has blamed others when things went wrong will now, no doubt, blame others for things lost, things misunderstood or tasks done less efficiently. A person who generally accepted life as it came will probably do the same when doing things becomes more challenging.

Perhaps the person most difficult to care for is the independent minded person who continues to insist they do things for themselves even when it is clear to the family they are not doing an adequate enough job to be safe or to ensure adequate nutrition and hygiene. This person may manipulate, deny difficulty, demand or blame others or things to stay in control of their own life. They will therefore resist any offer of assistance or advice.

Families may hear something like the following:

- "The toaster won't work anymore. It burns everything. I threw it out."

- "You didn't tell me that. Why did you leave me out of the plan?"

- "This coffee pot makes terrible coffee now. I don't know what is wrong with the way things are made these days."

- "I can do that myself; what are you doing, making me look stupid?"

- "I can still do the bills; I need to know how you are spending my money."

These responses are not easy to deal with.

My In-Laws: a Personal Story

Both my in-laws have had dementia. My father-in-law, who was a quiet, easygoing gentleman, took things in stride, even when he was diagnosed with Alzheimer's disease. I remember being with him when he was given the diagnosis. On the drive home, I said, "So, Dad, what do you make of that diagnosis?" He simply replied, "It wasn't what I wanted to hear, for sure, but we'll see." That was that! He rarely became angry at others' efforts to help him. This was his persona. He simply stopped doing things that became difficult for him. He became quieter, laughed less often and talked less.

My husband Curt would quiz him, feeling he was helping his father "exercise his brain," that if his dad tried hard enough, he would be able to recall the answer to the question posed. "Come on, Dad, you know. Think! If you use your brain, it will work longer." His father would just smile wanly and shake his head, not answering. That was back in the late 1980s. Knowing what he knows now, my husband feels sad about how he must have frustrated his dad. He lacked understanding of dementia and what his response should have been. (He wanted me to include this story so others would not feel the shame and guilt after the person is gone that he has.)

My mother-in-law, on the other hand, who is ninety-eight years old, responded to having dementia very differently. She was unaware of how changes in her ability and her behavior were impacting her life (and ours) and refused all attempts to care for her. She has expressed her frustration for the last ten years of dementia in anger towards anyone who implies she needs help with tasks or decision making. This has presented professional care partners and our family members with some real challenges. I should write a book on just our family's trials trying to care for her. I've documented our many efforts in a story on my computer called "The Move to Assisted Living," the beginning of our taking charge to keep her safe and well nourished. Some of those trials are in this book.

My mother-in-law has taught me much about working with resistant people! I tried many habilitation approaches with her and refined them as they failed or fell short of the expected outcome. I should thank her for being my best teacher of using habilitation approaches with resistant people! Using habilitation approaches has made many seemingly impossible situations work out.

A Word about Habilitation Therapy Approaches

The approaches in this book have a base in habilitation therapy. The habilitation approach in caring about and for someone with a diagnosis of dementia was developed by Paul Raia PhD and Joanne Koenig Coste M.Ed of the Massachusetts Alzheimer's Association. Joanne has written a fine book called Learning to Speak Alzheimer's, (published by Houghton Mifflin.)

A longitudinal research study that began in 1987 was conducted to see if the expected positive results from using habilitation approaches could be substantiated. This research was conducted at New York University School of Medicine Alzheimer's Disease Center, and the protocol and results are available in a book Counseling the Alzheimer's Caregiver by Mary S. Mittelman, Cynthia Epstein and Alicia Pierzchala (published by AMA Press in 2003.) It is written with teaching professionals in mind about how to counsel the caregiver, but the book can add to your knowledge of the dementia care partnering experience.

The research showed that when a care partner is educated in dementia care and given ongoing support by phone, the patient stays home a year or longer.

The habilitation approach in care partnering is designed to encourage successful participation in everyday life, and to give a person value, purpose and meaning. Learning these approaches is very satisfying to the carepartner as you see them bring comfort to the person you care for. Care partners I've taught habilitation approaches have all reported positive changes. Here are some of their comments from satisfaction surveys we've received.

- "I enjoy her more."

- "I talk differently and he responds differently, and seems happier. And I am, too."

- "I appreciate him more."

- "She seems calmer, happier, and so am I."

- "She actually enjoyed being bathed."

- "I changed my expectations of him. That made all the difference."

- "I had no idea what I do has so much impact on her."

- "I don't argue with him anymore. I never won anyway!"

- "I smile more these days."

- "We are touching more. It feels good. Now I can be his wife instead of his nursemaid. "

Habilitation approaches enhance life for the person with dementia, ease care partnering and keep relationships alive by creating a more cooperative spirit between care partners.

One goal of learning habilitation approaches to dementia-driven behaviors is to produce positive feelings for both the person with memory loss and the person caring for him. It brings both a feeling of empowerment. A second goal is to encourage continued participation in life by accommodating his difficulty doing things.

Coaching families helps us identify the challenges together and address them one by one. Each family finds some behaviors more challenging than others.

Pause for thought

What behavioral change as a result of dementia would be hard for you to deal with in your family member?

_____

_____

_____

_____

_____

Changing Isn't Always Easy

Dementia care is stressful for many reasons, but I believe the greatest stress (but eventual success) comes because we must change our responses from what we have practiced throughout the life of the relationship to something unfamiliar and therefore awkward at first. The longer people have been in a relationship, the more challenging it is to learn working together in a new way.

We generally want relationships to remain predictable. When a person behaves different from what we have come to expect, we are puzzled. If we learn the change is permanent, we become alarmed, sad or angry. When called to learn new responses, we feel tension.

None of us particularly likes change…unless, of course, we create it. For example, it is all right if we decide on a job change and turn in our letter of resignation, but if we receive a pink slip delivered to our desk, that is not! Being faced with caring for someone with memory loss, a change we didn't anticipate, requires a willingness and perseverance to adapt to the change.

What do families need and want? Families express the need to find ways to reduce their fears, frustrations and anger, and to feel more confident in caring for their family member. They want to become hopeful again and keep their stress under control. Practical needs are those of understanding what is happening to their family member, understanding how to respond more effectively to the changes in ability, how to provide safety and how to plan for the future.

Learning new responses to behavior is rewarding, albeit hard work; care partners feel more empowered as they see new, more productive or safer behaviors emerge. The person with dementia also feels more successful in the world and senses an easiness living with and being able to enjoy people.

What if I Don't Get Along with the Person I Care for?

Sometimes the care partner is not fond of, or actually dislikes, the person with dementia who they must care for. One care partner said, "When someone was asked to step forward to take on the care for Dad, it wasn't that I stepped forward; everyone else stepped back." Even in this difficult state of affairs it is still beneficial to learn habilitation approaches to make care easier. Helping the person with dementia to feel calm and experience more success in doing things brings a sense of well being to the carepartner. I've even seen conflicted relationships heal as the care partner develops compassion for his or her charge through the understanding of dementia behavior and the use of habilitation.

So, let's get started sharing in the lives of people, like you, who learned the habilitation approaches, and share in the changes it made for them. The final goal is to keep people in relationship throughout the journey of dementia.

If you are caring for someone with dementia you will see yourself in many of the stories. The principles are transferable; use them liberally! Develop your own approaches, but base them on the principles of habilitation.

Care Partnering: What Is It?

Let me speak about the term care partnering. The term caregiver indicates there is a "giver" of care and a "recipient" of that care. It does not denote a shared effort toward a goal. Care partnering speaks of working together, albeit in a new way: the habilitation way. Care partners accommodate the changes brought on by dementia by learning to speak differently, to respond differently and to work differently with their family member.

THE TEN CHALLENGES IN DEMENTIA CARE

Now you are ready to meet the challenges of caring for someone with dementia. You have learned what the brain does, what it can't do well when affected by dementia, and what behavior is all about. Some of the areas of challenge overlap, but if you are willing and a bit creative you can meet them all. Each challenge will be explained, and anecdotes will give examples of how the challenge was dealt with. The habilitation principles used in the solution to the challenge will be repeated at the end of the anecdote. These are all true stories of real people with names and some details changed to maintain privacy.

The ten challenges of care are to meet the changes in the following:

1. Memory and orientation
2. Attention and concentration
3. Mood regulation
4. Language
5. Activity
6. Safety
7. Care partner stress
8. Sexuality
9. Preserving self-esteem
10. Moving on: living in a new home

We'll take one at a time, discussing the area of challenge, some general guidelines for meeting the challenge and stories to illustrate using these approaches. Some will work for you; some will need to be adjusted to your partner's individual needs. Some will work one day and not the next! Prepare to be forgiving of your care partner and you as you learn.

Challenge #1:
MEMORY AND ORIENTATION

Memory

Memory loss is always a challenge for care partners. Repetitive questioning and telling stories over and over can be exhausting. The person with dementia may accuse his partner of leaving him out of plans because he has no memory of having been told.

"You never told me that?"

"Why are you always ignoring me?"

Or, he may argue that she did something that you know she forgot to do and needs to do.

"I did bathe. Don't say I didn't!"

"These clothes are clean; I just put them on this morning."

Remember, this is not forgetfulness; forgetfulness is normal.

Forgetfulness means it will be remembered later. We call that memory lapse. Memory loss, on the other hand, means the event was never stored in the brain; what isn't stored cannot be remembered.

Disorientation

There are different kinds of disorientation: time, place and person. This may be expressed by not knowing where you are, not knowing who you are, or not knowing the time, day, month or year. Time is confusing to the person experiencing these distortions. It is as if he is living in another time or in a place different from yours. He may not recognize himself in a mirror (this is generally later in the disease) or fail to recognize you for who you are. He also may think there are two of you, referring to you as if you are another person. He may not realize he is in his own home and express uneasiness, voicing a need to "go home."

Spatial disorientation is unawareness of where your body is in relation to other objects or people. People affected in the occipital lobe are often spatially disoriented. They may trip over an obstacle like a threshold sensing it is flat. They may lift their feet up high over the threshold as if it were at a foot high. This disability presents safety concerns.

Tips to help someone with memory and disorientation:

These often go hand in hand, so it seems practical and useful to work with them both.

- Inform more than question. Avoid quizzing, for example, "Do you remember what day it is today?" It is unkind.

- Tell her what day and season it is first thing in the morning. "Good morning; breakfast is ready. It is snowing again."

- Use a day calendar and large-faced clocks at eye level—visual cues.

- Conspicuously post a white eraser board with the day, date and perhaps a brief plan for the day written on the board. It might say:

    Monday, November 4th

Nancy comes: bath @ 9.

Jack is coming @ 11.

Then you don't have to say "Don't forget; Nancy comes today at nine."

One woman in the early stage of Alzheimer's devised a To Do list for herself so she'd know she'd done important tasks. Upstairs in the bathroom she had a check-off list naming tasks like brush teeth, shower, take medicines, make bed. Downstairs in the kitchen was another white board: walk the dog, meet Mildred for coffee, breakfast, lunch, make dinner and evening medicines. She found that doing this gave her confidence she had remembered everything.

- Introduce people by name and association. "Mom, Jack is on the phone. He wants to speak to his mom."

- Reorient after he naps. Often people think it is a new day upon awakening from a nap. "It is four o'clock, almost time for your favorite program on TV."

- If she misplaces something, help look for it. This minimizes her feeling suspicious or frustrated. Often people believe someone has taken something because they have no memory of having hidden it somewhere in order to be able to find it later.

- If he accuses you of taking what he has misplaced, do not argue the point or try logical explanation to correct his thinking. "Let's look for it together," would be a better response. If you had no idea you had put something away in a special place so you'd remember where it was, it is easy to see how you'd think someone had taken it.

- Avoid sharing plans. This is hard for people. We are used to planning with those we live with. But she will probably forget what the plan was and be left with an uneasy feeling that she's supposed to be doing something or going somewhere. She may refuse to go (even if it is something pleasurable) simply because of this increased anxiety. Instead, tell her just before you need to get ready. "We have an appointment. Let's get your coat." Decrease the time between when she is informed and when the event is to take place.

- Later on in the disease, you may have to tell him on the way there to minimize fretfulness.

- If she appears confused or anxious, ask if you can clear something up. "Is something bothering you?" "Can I help clear something up for you?" Notice both of these are simple yes or no questions.

- Listen for the emotion behind words and respond to that. "You look afraid. You are safe with me; I'll take care of things," is a good response.

- Often all that he wants is simple clarity, comforting or reassurance. It is frightening to be unaware of where you are or where you are going. "We are meeting Jill at Bobbie's house. We are almost there."

Learn How to Respond When a Person Is Disoriented

Anecdote—We're Not Married Anymore?

This is a story of Janet and Al who had enjoyed a fifty-two-year marital relationship based on trust and mutual respect. Al had never spoken an unkind word, according to Janet. I was called after an explosive incident in which Al ended up in a jail cell and Janet in an emergency room.

This is what had happened. Al woke up one morning, looked at Janet coming into the bedroom and demanded, "Where is Janet? What have you done to her?" Janet explained that she was his wife and proceeded to get their wedding photo and the fiftieth wedding anniversary photo taken just two years previously. He bellowed, "You're not my wife! You've hurt her, haven't you?" He proceeded to jump out of bed and hit her. She escaped with a cell phone into the bathroom and called 911. The police took the "offender" to jail and called an ambulance for the victim. Of course, Al didn't belong in jail, and when questioned, he denied the assault. He had no memory of having hit his wife.

Janet was treated and released to home within a few days; Al was brought to a mental health unit for evaluation. Then he was released home to her care. She wanted to take him home but didn't know if it was safe to do so. The assault was reported to protective service and I was called to teach Janet how to avoid this happening again.

Janet had to learn about fiblets. It felt deceitful for her to tell fiblets to Al since they had always dealt truthfully with one another. After much coaching she saw the potential value of fiblets. She agreed to try if he should not recognize her again, to say, "She went to the store for your favorite cinnamon raisin bread, and wanted me to tend the breakfast until she returns." She memorized this so she wouldn't panic.

Knowing that a person with dementia's inability to recognize family members is often a momentary thing, we counted on his feeling relieved that Janet was safe, on an errand to please him. This satisfied his immediate need to know his wife was safe. It worked. By the time Al was fully awake and came into the kitchen, he greeted a very uneasy Janet. "Well, good morning, Jan, what's for breakfast today?"

Janet learned that fiblets are useful to avoid harm and reduce her husband's fear based on unreal thinking.

- Fiblets are always used to benefit the person with dementia.

- Fiblets can be helpful to ensure safety for everyone.

- Agitation may be a response to the care partner's stress.

- Agitation may be a response to lack of understanding or fear. See discussion of causes for agitation on page [ ].

Anecdote—Lack of Recognition and Some Creative Solutions

Tom wanted some guidance about disturbing behaviors of his wife Bea. He obviously loved her deeply and was concerned and hurt over her lack of recognition of him at times. Occasionally, usually late afternoon, when he was watching television, Bea would come from another room and demand an explanation as to why he was watching her husband's TV.

"Who are you and why are you watching Tom's television?" She would get agitated, screaming at him to leave. He had tried explaining, to no avail, that he was her husband and that he lived here with her. Once she left the room to call the police. That particular time, he gave up trying to dissuade her and waited to see what would happen. When he finally entered the kitchen minutes later, she was happily doing something else, as if the incident had never happened. She turned around and began asking him what he wanted for dinner, showing no hostility whatever. He was baffled at this sudden change in mood.

Pause for thought

How would you handle this situation? Would you try to help her "understand"? If so, how would you do that?

_____

_____

_____

_____

_____

I explained to Tom that lack of recognition of a familiar person is often momentary. When he reported that when she left for the kitchen and moments later recognized him for who he was, that showed me she had immediate memory loss and could respond to a change in the emotional atmosphere.

We decided on the following tactic if she persisted in being angry with him and threatening him with a call to the police. He would say, "I'm sorry. I must have gotten the wrong house. I'll leave now."

Then I instructed him to slowly circle the outside of the house, enter the back door and announce, "Hi, Bea, it's Tom. I'm home!" She recognized him, as she had in the kitchen moments after the prior encounter in the living room. "Oh, I'm so glad you're home. I've been frightened. Don't leave me alone like that again! I need you here with me."

You can see how knowing Bea had immediate memory loss with some momentary disorientation led to a different response from Tom that resulted in removing the fear for her and the aggravation for Tom.

- Get into the person's sense of reality and work with them there.

- Avoid reorienting a person to your sense of reality.

- You can change a potentially explosive situation by satisfying the immediate need. For Bea, that was to feel safe. She didn't feel safe with this "stranger" in her house.

How to Ease the Lack of Recognition for Family and Friends

There is probably no more anticipated dread for a family than that time when their family member does not recognize them. It is a time of shock and a feeling of great loss. Even though a person with dementia may not recognize us, they do know that somehow we belong to them and will respond favorably if we adapt our approach and responses. Stating your name and your relationship to them helps them become oriented.

"Hi, Mom, it's me John. Is your day going well?"

Now she knows you're related to her even though she couldn't tell you how when you arrived. She may have shown recognition of your presence and been unable to identify you apart from others.

As family or visitor we have to be satisfied with lack of special recognition. Retrieving information from memory banks is very difficult, sometimes impossible for them. The person may also have a hard time attending to one event happening when the surroundings are busy. Identifying yourself makes it easier for them to attend to you.

- Identifying yourself and your relationship to them helps get on with the conversation.

- Disorientation can be momentary, and is rarely permanent.

- Awareness of surroundings lessens as dementia progresses.

- Paying attention in a busy environment is more difficult, perhaps impossible, for a person with dementia.

Anecdote—The Move to Assisted Living

This story is about my mother-in-law Betty's memory loss, persistent disorientation and lack of logic.

Betty moved to an assisted living residence as it became apparent she was getting confused and fearful living on her own. My husband Curt moved some of her favorite furniture and belongings and replicated the apartment as close to what it was at her home. She quickly adapted with familiar things surrounding her. Thinking she was on vacation, she began enjoying the socializing and the good meals. Eating more nutritious foods than when she lived alone, she improved in cognition and strength. (The brain needs good nutrition to work.)

Memory, however, was poor, both for immediate past events and for remote past events. She thought her parents were paying for this "vacation" and she needed to return home. She imagined her parents (both had died forty-five years before) were also vacationing there on another floor and that she needed to include them in all her social activities outside the "resort." She worried about the expense, even though she agreed it was a wonderful gesture to move her furniture there for her vacation!

Betty, an only child, born one year after her mother had a still-born son, had always been a companion to her mother through her growing up. She developed a feeling of responsibility for her mother's happiness. Trying to get her to go out for the evening was a challenge. She insisted her mother had to come, too.

When we wanted to take her out to dinner, she would fret that her mother needed to be invited. Curt encouraged her to leave a note for her mother. She wrote a note, promptly "forgot" she had, and again wanted to write a note telling her mother where she was going. She often took up to an hour to get organized and agree to leave with him. Memory disappeared in the throes of her anxiety.

The more anxious she became about her mother, the more disorganized she became. Often her agitation resulted in refusing to go with him at all. I suggested that he make up a few notes (she had written many) and carry one or two with him. The note could say, "Mother, we are at the 99 Restaurant. You are invited to meet us there." Each time she wanted to write a note, he would lift up the note and say, "Here is your note. We'll leave it at the front desk so she'll get it as soon as she arrives home." This sped up her getting ready for the dinner out.

Betty was living in another time in her mind. She often mistook Curt for her husband, having no memory of her deceased husband and their marriage of sixty years. She would look at her husband's picture and say, "I think I met him a long time ago. He was a likeable man. Mother liked him." Curt couldn't understand this and would try to help her remember his father. She would get agitated and called him a liar. "He is not dead; you're here!"

Curt was finally able to find some humor in being her "husband" when, one evening as we were driving away from her residence, she looked back over her shoulder (she sat in the front seat with her "husband" when we went out) and asked, "Couldn't you find a beau to accompany you tonight?" I said, "Well it was short notice. Do you mind if I tag along with you and Curt?" "No, not at all, dear, as long as you know he is going home with me!" "Absolutely!" I said, grinning at Curt's reflection in the rearview mirror.

- Satisfy the immediate need of the person with dementia in order to gain their cooperation.

- Each person's immediate need will be different, and satisfied differently. For Betty, it was to include her mother, whom she felt responsible for.

- Get into the person's reality and stay there with them.

- People need to feel in charge of what happens to them.

- People must feel they have choices.

Anecdote—Sometimes Some Humor Can Come from Disorientation

Maintaining a sense of humor is critical. Randy often didn't recognize his wife Deidre but enjoyed her company nonetheless. While riding with her to the day program, he would start to talk about his wife Deidre to his "friend" James. James was a long deceased friend of Randy's and, in his mind, the person who was driving him today. He would have a conversation "man to man" about women in general and Deidre in particular.

At first Deidre was alarmed and annoyed he didn't acknowledge her presence, but she had learned in our coaching not to try to reorient him. She began to enjoy the discussion (usually one-sided—his side) in good humor. Randy often told James how he loved Deidre and the funny things she did to make him laugh. To Deidre this became endearing, a new way of relating that was reminiscent of the relationship they had enjoyed when he was well. His emotions were exposed. and she enjoyed it. She never did figure out, however, how he could look at her and call her James. (She is a very attractive woman.)

"Oh, well, at least I know he loves me. He tells James all the time!" she said, laughing.

- Giving up personal need for recognition may lead to some interesting new information.

- Avoid reality orienting a person with dementia; enter their reality.

Anecdote—Handling Repetitive Questions

Here is another situation in which repetition due to memory loss is handled very nicely. Repetitious questions are often for lack of ability to initiate conversation that is meaningful.

Ann visited her mother, Dorothy, at the nursing home dementia unit where she had resided for six months. She dreaded visiting, knowing she would be asked the same three questions over and over. "How is business?" "How many people do you employ?" and "Are you making money?" Dorothy had owned her own successful business and was attuned to the importance of making a good living by employing many people to do the work. Ann would answer these questions perhaps fifty times in a one hour visit and looked for any excuse to leave. She felt badly about her reluctance to visit her mother. Ann needed a new strategy to deal with the repetitious questions.

I discovered that Dorothy had a severe attention deficit and was unable to attend to two things simultaneously. She could not sustain meaningful conversation. Dorothy was reverting to a subject she understood: work. She also had immediate memory loss and did not know she had asked these questions before.

Pause for thought

Think of reactionary (knee-jerk) behavior of yours you'd like to change to a more effective one.

_____

_____

_____

_____

_____

I suggested that Ann come to visit with a plan to do something with her mother. I asked her what activities interested her mother in the past. "She dabbled in drawing and painting after she sold her business and retired." Apparently Dorothy had really enjoyed this activity.

So, to limit the need for conversation, we decided Ann would bring a favorite food along with a drawing activity. She came armed with coffee and muffins and an art project that her mother could do with help. Ann had found a velvet-backed outline of a subject that, when colored in, resulted in a colorful picture. Knowing her mother liked cats and flowers, she chose one with flowers and kittens playfully batting at butterflies. I told Ann that interest and attention to the activity wouldn't be sustained unless she did the project with her mother, so Ann initiated talk by introducing the project while putting the coffee and muffin in front of her mother.

It was amazing! Dorothy hummed softly as she filled in the spaces with color, munching from time to time on a muffin and sipping her coffee. She asked only once about work, and Ann quickly redirected her by talking about the project they were doing. Now each time Ann visits she brings an activity and is enjoying her time with Dorothy much more.

- Focusing on a familiar activity may reduce repetitious questions.

- A person with dementia cannot easily attend to two activities at once.

- Activity won't be sustained if the person is left alone; do the activity with them.

Anecdote- Gotta feed the horse!

In past years, Jake had helped feed a friend Ed's horse. Ed had worked the late shift and had appreciated Jake tending to this late afternoon feeding. Jake enjoyed visiting the stable, which was about two miles from home, each day at four when his workday at the post office was done.

Jake now has dementia with severe memory loss. Living in the past he insisted he needed to go to the stable to feed the horse. His wife Ida tried to tell him the horse was sold long ago and that there was no need for him to go to the stable.

"It is empty. The horse is gone."

Jake would get very angry, punch his fists into his palms and call her names.

"Give me the keys to the car."

"You're jealous of a horse?"

Ida was becoming frightened of him and dreaded afternoons. She would sometimes try to ignore his behavior and leave to go for a walk, hoping he'd forget he wanted to go to the stable. This sometimes worked, but more often afternoons turned into a fighting match of words. Jake's perseverance on this subject was troublesome.

Pause for thought

What would you do to get Jake to stop demanding to go feed the horse?

_____

_____

_____

_____

_____

Asking Ida about Jake's current abilities, I learned he was having trouble doing common, everyday tasks. He could not figure out how to use the phone any longer. I also learned that he gave up on a task he could not do instead of asking for help. Jake had never once acknowledged his memory problems; also, he historically could not ever admit he was wrong or unable to do anything. His inability was not expressed in frustration; he merely gave up the activity.

The challenge was to distract him by giving him a task he couldn't perform. When he asked for the keys to the car to go to the stable to feed the horse, I told Ida to say she'd go look for them and for him to call Ed to see if he wanted Jake to feed the horse today. While she "looked" for the keys in another part of the house, taking her time, Jake would attempt to call Ed. (Ed had moved away ten years ago, and had sold the horse at that time.)

When Jake couldn't figure out how to use the phone, he quickly gave up, stating, "Oh, forget it." He'd sit back down in front of the television. Other times Ida would say, "You had the keys last. I don't know where you put them. Why don't you look for them while I go to the bathroom and spruce up?" Both these strategies were successful most days! He would give up looking for the keys, probably unable to sustain memory of what he was looking for, and she would stay in the bathroom an extra long time.

When even these approaches didn't work to satisfy him, Ida would take a short walk and hope the memory of what he wanted to do would fade and he would resume watching television. She always had tapes of his favorite team (the Red Sox—winning, of course) to pop in to entertain him!

- It is important to understand the person's coping style for new approaches to work.

- Learning that Jake had "never been wrong in his life" made designing an approach easier.

- Learning that he could no longer use a telephone was useful as well in designing approaches.

A side note: Television is not the activity of choice for the person with dementia! Unless it is an interactive show that will prompt participation, television is mind numbing. A mind needs stimulation to build new neural pathways. Jake needed a structured, interactive day, which he could have had at an adult day program. He is now residing in a dementia unit where he has found stimulation and a sense of belonging and safety.

Challenge #2:
ATTENTION AND CONCENTRATION

Processing of information is slowed, and holding on to it is difficult in the damaged brain; thus attention and concentration are impaired. Knowing this deficit, we must accommodate by helping the person focus on a task.

Anecdote—Where Are We? Egypt?

Joan's inability to attend was the most severe I'd ever seen. She sat nearby as Tom and I talked about their planned trip to northern Africa. I was concerned about Joan wandering away from him when he couldn't keep his eyes on her every moment. It wouldn't be that she wanted to wander away; it would be that she couldn't maintain attention long enough to realize she was traveling with him.

Her eyes roamed the room as we talked that day, unable to attend to the conversation. The ceiling fan distracted her, as did the rubbish trucks on the street outside the window, causing her to jerk her attention first one way, then another. I tried to bring her into the conversation, maintaining eye contact. As soon as an extraneous noise or vision attracted her, I lost her attention.

This would be a troublesome, potentially unsafe deficit in a foreign country where perhaps few spoke English. I asked her if she would know what to do if she became lost in Egypt. She said she'd go looking for Tom. I asked if she knew who could help her find Tom. She looked blankly and repeated, "I'd look for Tom." The lack of attention and concentration as well as a lack of logic in problem solving made the trip a potential danger to Joan wandering and getting lost. If he decided to travel, I suggested a Safe Return bracelet and that he update the SR information on the central computer to include his being out of the country and to have a written itinerary left for his children.

- Prepare ahead when in new surroundings; it may make a person much more confused.

- A person with dementia usually becomes confused in new situations or places.

- The Safe Return Program of the Alzheimer's Association is available at 888-572-8566. This program supplies the care recipient with a small bracelet with a code on the back that matches information kept on a central computer. It relays the whereabouts of family members, important medication and home address.

Anecdote—Lack of Ability to Attend Saved this Coach's Hide!

I was coaching a man who had no one to stay with his wife while we talked. This was our first coaching session; my usual request at this time is that the person with dementia be elsewhere to avoid embarrassment hearing a family member talk about their condition and its impact on them. But this time, the man's diagnosed wife sat just to my right in a chair set against the wall. Her husband and I were at the dining room table.

As the session progressed I became aware of building tension in her body. From the corner of my eye, I noted her rubbing the chair arms, tightening up her facial muscles and finally clenching the arm of the chair with a strong grip. She was getting very agitated, and I was the trigger. There is always a trigger for any behavior; behavior is goal directed. Although she probably didn't understand much of the conversation we were having, she did understand it was about something that upset her husband. She was responding to the strained emotional atmosphere surrounding the discussion.

Counting on her memory loss, I turned to her saying, "You've been so patient while we jabbered away here. Your husband has been talking about what a wonderful wife you've been to him for the last forty-four years." I saw her body visibly relax some; she unclenched her hands and laid them in her lap. I proceeded, "Would you mind if I came again and we could talk woman to woman?" I waited for her response.

"Sure, I'd like that. Do you have to go so soon? You just got here." I'd been there one and a half hours. She followed me to the door smiling and waved as I drove away in the car.

- Mood is contagious. Mirror the mood you want to evoke.

- Count on short attention span to help the strategy work.

- Do not talk negatively about a person in front of them without expecting a negative reaction.

- Avoid talking about a person's disturbing behavior in front of them.

Anecdote—Mirroring: a Visual Prompt to Change Behavior

Anne called me when she was "at her wits end" dealing with her husband Ed's annoying behaviors. He walked about the house with a coffee mug, splashing coffee all over the floors. He also was beginning to eat inappropriately, tearing apart his food and putting odd mixtures together. It sickened her and she didn't want to eat with him any longer. These behaviors were compounded for her due to the existing conflict they'd had throughout their thirty-five year marriage. She had always "taken care" of him, and now it was simply more of the same. Her patience with him was short.

The first problem was easily solved with a covered coffee mug from the local donut shop.

- When we are in the throes of change, we often react emotionally and don't see easy solutions.

Then I asked where they ate meals. She showed me a long parson's table parallel to a blank white wall. She stated they ate sitting side by side, facing the wall. I suggested he might need a visual prompt to eat more appropriately and that if she sat opposite, mirroring how to eat, he might follow her example. She agreed to try this and, sure enough, he began to eat more appropriately.

- Mirroring a desired behavior can be very effective in accommodating lost abilities.

- Lack of stimulation (the blank wall; the lack of conversation) may make a person more confused.

Challenge #3:
MOOD REGULATION

The frontal lobe is often involved in Alzheimer's dementia, making it hard to keep mood stable. We can help, however, by responding differently to the emotion expressed. Staying actively involved in daily life helps regulate mood as well. We are generally happier when doing things that are pleasurable to us. It is the same for those with dementia.

Irritability, as well as rummaging and fidgeting, are often signs of confusion. It is not helpful to point out the confusion, but clearing up the confusion can help. Rummaging should be allowed. Put away important items you don't want to have rummaged through and perhaps lost. A locked file cabinet for valuables is a good idea one man used. His wife had rummaged through papers and often hidden them to keep them "safe." Once they were safely locked up, he didn't worry so about her rummaging and often supplied her with unimportant papers to sort for him.

In some dementias like frontal temporal dementia or Pick's disease, an inability to regulate mood is a hallmark symptom. Mood is regulated in the frontal lobe as we said in Step #1, and if damaged cannot perform that function. These people may fly off the handle, scream, curse, behave unpredictably or become aggressive. It is most important for these folks to be in as stable and quiet an environment as possible. This is not ever easy in a family setting.

Being delusional or experiencing visual hallucinations is another cause for a change in mood. When the delusion is one of a paranoid nature or the hallucination is frightening, it is no wonder the person responds in fear. The fear is expressed in anger, blaming, suspiciousness, irritability and aggression.

Sometimes the person may direct all the rage at one other person— usually the caregiver. If the rage cannot be controlled with behavioral approaches or an antipsychotic medication, this is often the reason for seeking long-term placement in a dementia unit.

Most times, however, mood can be modified with a change in our behavioral response or with an adjustment in the environment. We will look at changes in mood under other challenges as well, but generally the mood is one of fear, anger or a result of confusion. We can learn to relieve our care partners of the resulting feelings.

Anecdote—The Devil Made Me Do It!

This is an example of an elder whose anger was sudden and intense, the accompaniment of delusional thinking. I was speaking with the client Bernadette's two daughters. It was our first coaching visit, and Bernadette's son Douglas was unable to take Bernadette for a drive during our visit as planned. This meant Bernadette sat in on our conversation, a situation I try hard to avoid.

Making sure to keep the visit as social and non-threatening as possible, I kept my folder of teaching materials out of sight. Thankfully, Bernadette was very hard of hearing, but she sensed uneasiness in our conversation in spite of my frequent smiles in her direction. One of her daughters picked up and opened the folder, revealing a picture of the brain that I use to I explain brain function. Bernadette asked, "What is that?" Trying to soften my answer, I said, "A head." One daughter corrected me, saying to her mother, "It is a brain." "Oh, I don't have one of those anymore." retorted Bernadette, not without some sadness in her voice. Directly after that she turned to me and said, "You are a devil from Satan. You've been here at least three hours! I want you to leave now!"

----- *Pause for thought* -----

What should I do in this situation?

_____

_____

_____

_____

_____

Bernadette's daughters were embarrassed, reporting she had said something similarly aggressive to a niece recently.

I answered Bernadette, "You are right. I've overstayed my welcome and you need to eat dinner. Thank you for your hospitality. I shall leave you now." The folder was put aside and closed. I approached Bernadette, who was seated, thanking her while holding her hand in mine and bending to eye level. Immediately she smiled and whispered, "I'm kidding you." And she winked at me. Then she saw me to the door, smiling, telling me to bundle up against the cold.

Bernadette had not been kidding when she said I was a devil from Satan. She had been frightened by the picture of the brain. As a visual cue, it evoked fear, perhaps about her awareness of her confusion . I had to relieve her fear by changing the mood. In this way, I didn't respond to her words, but to her emotion, restoring a more favorable mood. I made sure not to set another appointment in her earshot. We made plans for future meetings via email later that evening. I was also able to remind her daughters of looking beyond words to the emotion expressed. Relieve the anxiety by removing the trigger than evoked it. Then change the mood by responding instead of reacting to the words. Mood can change by meeting the need expressed.

- Look beyond the words spoken to the emotion being expressed.

- If you are aware of the trigger for the negative emotion, remove it. In this case it was the picture of the brain and me!

- Respond to a behavior; avoid reacting.

Reassure the Person of His Worth to You

I often hear from families by phone and e-mail asking for advice about immediate challenges. A few evenings ago I received a phone call from a woman I had never met. She began by saying the day had been very disturbing; her husband told her he was not taking his heart medicine for angina any more.

"I've been told I am going to die soon and I won't need it where I'm going," he had told her.

I asked how often he usually took the medicine.

"Not often, but he says he is going to die. He won't eat, either. What should I do? I asked him who told him this, that it was ridiculous. He couldn't hear that; I think he may be seeing things again."

"Don't try logic with him," I reminded her. "If he is in a delusional state, he thinks what he believes to be true is real. Sometimes what a person says is not the main issue. What do you think he is saying? What does he want to hear from you?" I asked.

"Is he afraid of dying, do you think?"

"I don't know either of you personally yet, but you might try letting him know you need him and will be very lost without him," I suggested.

"Okay, I'll try that," she said and hung up.

The next morning I called her back to ask how it went. She said,

"I went to the bed where he was laying, waiting to die. I lay down beside him, rubbed his back and told him I was going to miss him terribly."

"So what happened?"

"He got up and ate pizza with me! What made that change things?"

"You satisfied his need; he wanted your expression of love. He needed to know you still needed him and would miss him."

- Fear finds its expression in behavior.

- Delusions and hallucinations are expressions of concern.

Anecdote—Be Gentle with the Colonel

Another time I was visiting with the wife of a retired colonel in the Air Force. She had requested help to deal with her husband's anger toward her when she spent time with others. She had had to call 911 a few times when his aggressiveness became frightening, but she was reluctant to consider him living elsewhere.

As we spoke quietly he slept by a window. I noticed he was dressed in many layers of clothing, ill-suited to the warm weather. He was also unshaven and looked dirty. She concurred that he hadn't washed in many weeks nor had he changed his clothing.

He awoke while I was there and, after glaring at me from the doorway to the living room, came and stood over me, menacingly clenching his fists. I turned to him and said that I had overstayed my welcome and indicated this by picking up my coat. He backed up but continued clenching his fists and looking angry. I thanked him for having me and out of habit being polite, held out my hand to shake his. He took my hand in a death grip. Okay, I thought, how do I get out of this? I decided that to pull away would be a mistake, so I just put my free hand on top of his and said, "My, you are strong. I certainly am glad you are a military officer who treats ladies with respect." At that, he stood tall and saluted me. I smiled for a few reasons as I left the house.

On the way to the car, I reminded his wife to call 911 any time he became aggressive and to consider looking into a living residence that could handle his anger.

- Appeal to the positive side of an angry person.

- Do not panic, pull away, and struggle with an angry person.

- Anger is generally a result of fear, paranoid ideation, frustration, possessiveness of the caregiver or damage to the part of the brain that controls impulse.

Challenge #4:
LANGUAGE

Learning to speak in a new way is a work in progress. It means the care partner must have uncommon common sense. Once you appreciate that the brain is not allowing the person to comprehend his environment or express his response to that difficulty, you will speak in a different way based on this on this newly acquired information. A decline in the ability to use and understand language is common in Alzheimer's. The hippocampus isn't retaining what is said, the temporal lobes are not processing it quickly and retrieving language is slowed. We manage our lives through our speech. This is a hard loss.

When speaking to someone with language deficits, I speak in the same way I do with someone with English as a second language. I enunciate, maintain eye contact, speak more slowly and simply and avoid complex sentences, questions and subjects.

In speaking with people with language problems due to dementia, we must ask ourselves some questions. What does the person need at this moment? What is she trying to express? We must accommodate her deficit.

- Always state the person's name before speaking. This gains her attention. People with dementia always have attention deficits.

- Maintain eye contact with her through the entire conversation.

- If you lose eye contact, touch her forearm gently and reengage her.

- Keep language simple and slow; avoid complexity.

- Avoid speaking from another room or from behind. Come to the front. She may forget you are in the room and be startled, misunderstand you and experience frustration or irritability.

- Keep noise to a minimum (turn off radios, TVs, dishwashers, etc.) when speaking.

- Limit conversation to one person speaking at a time.

- If you've lost her, repeat what the conversation is about. This will help her "catch up" and feel included again. (Persons with dementia complain of being left out and often get angry when they feel this way. "I feel ignored," said one man.)

- Use closed-ended questions: ones that can be answered with yes or no. Complex questions are too hard to process.

- Ask questions that offer a choice of no more than two things, i.e., instead of asking, "What do you want to eat?" say, "It is lunch. Do you want tuna or egg sandwich with your soup?"

- Avoid questions that ask what, when, where, who, how and especially why. She especially won't know why she did something. Instead try to discover the intent of the behavior.

- Use visual cues more than words. People with cognitive impairment respond more easily to visual prompts. They lose comprehension and don't understand explanation.

- Visual prompts "remind" the brain what to do.

- Avoid switching subjects. It is too hard for her to follow.

- If she has trouble finding a word, and you think you know it, supply it. "Is sweater the word you are looking for?"

- If she uses the wrong word, do not correct her. It only points out her disability.

Assisting the person with language problems can be as easy as supplying the word he can't find. Retrieval of information, which is slowed, makes talking to others more difficult. Quizzing a person with twenty questions to lead them to the word is unkind. The brain is not allowing him to "find" the word.

I met a woman beginning to have trouble finding words and using the correct word for an object. As we were speaking and it was apparent she was struggling with language, I started supplying her with words, as it was evident to me what she was trying to say. I asked her, "Do you mind my giving you words or is it annoying?"

"Oh no" she replied, "it is very helpful. Can you tell my son to stop making me try to find a word? He keeps telling me if I try hard enough I'll remember the word. He says I have to exercise my brain! It is so embarrassing; I feel like a fool. And I get angry at him. I don't want that, but he makes me out to be crazy. Sometimes I don't want him around me."

The frustration of aphasia: Aphasia is an inability to use and/or understand language. It is common in certain conditions like stroke, and in frontal-temporal lobe dementia.

Anecdote—We're Fire and Water—Always Have Been!

Lila and Murray were arguing many times daily. Although their marriage had always been "fire and water," as he described it, conflict had recently increased. Murray had had a stroke a year ago, which left him with aphasia (difficulty processing language). He did not comprehend what others were saying and had a hard time expressing his ideas as well. He would get so agitated when frustrated that he would throw things against the wall in anger and call Lila terrible names.

I was concerned that his lack of judgment when angry would result in Lila being injured. Lila was very hard of hearing but had recently received two hearing aids, which she complained "made things too loud." As a result she talked more softly and Murray would further misunderstand her.

When he didn't respond to her questions, she accused him of ignoring her. In speaking with them both, the language challenge was unmistakable. When Lila and I were talking, Murray would become irritated and yell, "I don't know what you are saying! What are you contriving against me?"

When I spoke to him I used simple, concrete language, talking as I would perhaps with someone just learning English. I maintained consistent eye contact, waited for what I had said to be processed, repeated myself if his facial expression told me he didn't understand and waited for him to express himself. Even with that, it was sometimes too frustrating for him to keep up. He would then revert to perseverating about something irritating to him. His reasoning was often lacking in logic entirely.

Murray was unable to stay in contact with the conversation, and Lila was unwilling to accommodate his disability. Both needed time away from one another to lessen the toxic situation. Their daughter Amy arranged to have Lila picked up to attend the senior center, and a male companion trained in working with people like Murray was hired. He understood how to relate in light of Murray's language deficits.

• Some challenges are best resolved by separating antagonists!

- Expressive aphasia (inability to say what you want to say) is very frustrating for a person.

Anecdote—Using Language to Change Behavior

Marion was terrified of her recent memory loss and confusion. She was a chronically anxious, depressed woman. When she found something difficult to understand, she would ask her daughter Rita to "explain" it to her. When an answer was given, Marion would become angry with frustration; she was unable to process the answer, so she asked another question and another, which exhausted her daughter. Rita had tried answering every question as completely as she could, but this would just make Marion angrier. She would yell, "I've never been so hated in my whole life!"

Rita had been her mother's emotional supporter for her lifetime, soothing, comforting and listening to her when Marion was upset about something. Now her attempts to comfort or clarify were rejected, seen as ways to deliberately frustrate Marion. Thus, Marion felt hated!

It was important that Rita develop short answers and strategies to reduce her mother's frustration, thereby avoiding or minimizing accusations. Giving short concrete answers to her questions helped. If Marion became dissatisfied with the short answer, her daughter could say, "That's all I know." Rita was able reduce her mother's agitation and relieve herself of feeling that she failed to comfort her mother.

I instructed Rita to respond to Marion's accusation of being hated without "explanation." She agreed to avoid refuting that statement, understanding it was her mother's way to express her fear of failing. She agreed to say, "It must feel terrible to feel like that."

- Satisfy the immediate emotional need, in this case to successfully accomplish tasks.

- Avoid the use of logic and reason. It cannot be processed and will add to frustration.

- Avoid long explanations; they are not helpful.

- Develop simple responses to repetitive accusations that acknowledge the feeling expressed, but don't defend yourself. These responses may have to be scripted and memorized.

Challenge #5:
ACTIVITY

Maintain Pleasurable, Meaningful Activities Through Adaptation and Structure

It is imperative to engage a person with dementia in as much of his own care and in family activities as often as possible. Activity reduces confusion, restlessness, apathy and psychiatric signs like delusion, hallucinations and paranoia. Activity provides structure, purpose and meaning to life. When lacking initiative and interest abilities due to dementia, a person may resort to retreating to bed or to the television, neither of which are activities that lend to brain stimulation. We must accommodate them by setting up activity. However, no one can structure each day all day; an adult day program can help. Adult programs offer activities suited to the person's current ability. This assures success, uses up energy and provides social interaction for people who cannot do that for themselves.

Anecdote—Keep on Dancing!

Miriam and Tom had always loved dancing. In spite of Miriam's progressing dementia, she was still able to dance up a storm. It was a Saturday night ritual Tom wanted to continue. It was fun, Miriam was in an element she loved and they spent time with friends. The problem was that Miriam often ended up in bed instead of dressing to go out! The challenge was to discover why she went to bed instead of going dancing.

I asked Tom to tell me how he asked Miriam. We looked at this together step by step to find out where the glitch was.

"I get ready first and tell her to get ready. I put out a dressy dress, and go downstairs while she is dressing. Every time lately when I go up after twenty minutes, I find her in bed, in her pajamas instead of a dressed." "What happens then?" I asked. "I yell at her. 'What are you doing in bed? Don't you want to go dancing?' She gets upset, starts to cry and the night is spoiled. This is happening every Saturday night.

"Then she confronts me the next day, 'When are we going out dancing again? You never ask me any more.' I explain we didn't because she went to bed instead. She denies this and says I just don't want to dance with her anymore. Another argument ensues."

Miriam has immediate memory loss. She is a determined woman who likes to be appreciated and responds to criticism by blaming. She also has a problem with time disorientation, being unable to tell whether it has been an hour or a minute since something transpired. She responds to visual cues in the environment. We determined that Miriam couldn't hold onto the offer to get dressed in private, so half-way up the stairs she was unsure what she was going there for. Entering the bedroom, the bed was a visual cue to "tell" her what she was going upstairs for. It was getting dark outside as well. Ignoring the dress on the chair, she prepared herself for sleep.

Pause for thought

How would you help Tom and his wife to continue to go dancing?

_____

_____

_____

_____

We developed this plan. Tom would dress in the bedroom at the same time Miriam did so she had the visual cue of what she was preparing for. He would tell her she looked beautiful in each of two appropriate dresses he had hanging in view, and then ask her which one she would wear for him. "You look great in both. Will you wear one for me tonight?" She chose one and continued to dress with Tom mirroring the task on the other side of the bed. As they dressed, he talked simply and quietly about how they both enjoyed dancing. I suggested he might have dancing music playing in the room to further prompt her and keep her relaxed. With this plan implemented each week, Tom and Miriam continued to go dancing on Saturday nights.

- Mirroring a task helps the person with dementia stay on the task and complete it. (Seeing the items needed to get ready and seeing Tom getting ready were the visual cues Miriam needed to be successful.)

- Give people choices whenever possible. (This avoids using controlling measures which are seldom, if ever, received well.)

- Create a desire to choose by making it beneficial to them. (Tom told Miriam she looked smashing in either dress and kept it romantic rather than controlling.)

Anecdote—Visual Cueing for Toileting Success

Edyth was a very bright woman who at eighty-two was diagnosed with early Alzheimer's disease. She enjoyed classical music that soothed her in the late afternoon when she became restless and sometimes irritable. Edyth had spatial disorientation, getting turned around in her home of thirty years. This presented a toileting challenge as she wandered about the apartment looking for the bathroom and frequently got there too late. Incontinence became a real concern for the young daughter who lived upstairs. She would often find puddles of urine just outside the door of the bathroom. Having two small children, the daughter was becoming irritated about this added task each morning.

Pause for thought

Think of some reasons Edyth may be incontinent.

_____

_____

_____

_____

_____

Counting on Edyth's incontinence being caused by her failure to find the bathroom, we left only the light in the bathroom on at night, and put reflective foot imprints on the floor from the side of her bed to the bathroom. This worked for some time with success. One night someone left the light on in the kitchen, where the floor is the same color as the bathroom floor. In the morning there was the familiar puddle in the middle of the kitchen. Everyone made sure the kitchen light was out each night thereafter!

Later in the disease, Edyth was unable to figure out what to do once she found the bathroom. Figuring out how to use the toilet became the challenge. Since she still comprehended written language, a sign was posted over the toilet saying TURN AROUND. On the opposing wall the sign said SIT DOWN. This helped her use the toilet with some measure of success for a while longer. Notice the progression of visual cues to aide a person to perform personal tasks for themselves.

•Never think incontinence is a progression of the disease without checking out other reasons first.

•Incontinence can be caused by confusion, spatial disorientation or sequencing difficulty (taking clothes off and manipulating items needed for toileting).

Anecdote—There Is More Than One Way to Bathe a Woman!

One husband approached bathing resistance a bit dramatically. His wife was very resistant to showering. Each day as she sat at the kitchen table after breakfast, he'd walk by with a small bucket of warm water, "tripping" as he approached her and spilling the water over her. She would jump up saying, "I'm all wet. I'm cold!" He'd offer to help her out of her clothes (he had the shower all prepared to help her "warm up"). He had read about the changes in the brain and the resulting behaviors. He knew not to try to coerce her or try to reason with her about the need for hygiene. He found his own "solution" to the problem (no pun intended).

* Be creative in solving seemingly impossible situations.

* Look for reasons a person may resist showering. •(Looking at their bathroom, I was struck by the busyness of the wallpaper and wondered if the wife just felt lost in the bathroom. The wallpaper was a dark green jungle print, which might have been intriguing when she was well but was very confusing for her now.)

Anecdote—Enough Carrots for a Week!

This is a personal story that makes me smile each time I think about it. My mother in law, Elizabeth, who has a progressive dementia, always wants to feel helpful. When she visited with us at the beginning of her disease, she would ask over and over, "What can I do to help you prepare dinner?" I couldn't lure her to sit and simply keep me company, in spite of a drink and a snack to occupy her. She wanted a task. She had always loved serving a dinner with the table set "a la Martha Stewart"!

I decided I'd ask her to grate carrots for the top of the salad. It would occupy her time, keep her engaged and avoid my having to listen to her repetitious request for something to do. I set out the grater and a package of carrots on the island counter behind where I was tending the stove.

She began to hum and seemed satisfied with the task. After a time I turned around to see how she was doing. She stood behind a pyramid of grated carrots six inches high. I had to laugh at myself; I'd forgotten to set up the task in a way that she would understand what was wanted. We had enough carrots grated for salads for the week! I should have given her only as many carrots as she needed to grate to top the salad. We had a good laugh together. I don't think she understood what the joke was, but she did understand she had amused me.

- Doing something may reduce shadowing and repetitive questioning.

- Set up tasks to promote success.

This observation led to my further understanding how to set up tasks that would promote success.

In the beginning of Elizabeth's illness, I could simply tell her where the dishes and silverware were and how many of us there would be and she could do it well. Later on, I'd take the items out of the cabinet and point to the table. Instead of asking her to set the table and create a problem for her, I'd put out the correct number of plates, forks, knives and spoons. This reduced her need to decide how many and what to put on the table. She did well with that for a while, too. Later she had forgotten how to set a table, so I set up one place setting to cue her how to set the others. Much later, this wasn't enough structure. We set it together with step by step instruction and affirmation of a job well done. It took longer, yes. It also gave her delight in helping me serve dinner. The time was worth it for her and for me, too. If she didn't have a task, she would have been repeatedly asking how she could help.

- Setting up a task can provide meaningful activity for the person with memory loss.

- Adjust your expectations to fit the person's current ability.

Anecdote—Structure Ensures a Successful Day

Sarah had been a professional dancer, well known and adored by her fans. Now she suffered from confusion, memory loss, lack of judgment and mood regulation. She often complained she was ignored and disregarded. Her daughter Diane was tired of her accusations of being disregarded, and of her lack of appreciation. Diane said Sarah had demanded attention her whole life and had been accommodated by everyone, inside and outside the family. It seemed no amount of attention was enough to satisfy her now. Sarah had developed no hobbies, as her career had absorbed her.

Sarah had frontal lobe damage and could no longer initiate activity that was satisfying. She depended on everyone else to structure her time…but on her schedule!

Understanding that Sarah's brain wasn't allowing her to think up things to fill her day and that her lack of activity was contributing to her irritability and aggressive behavior (she had thrown over a chair in reaction to feeling ignored), we talked about activities that might be helpful. Others had to be engaged in this venture so it wouldn't fall on Diane to do it all. Diane's thirteen-year-old son agreed to play a game with Sarah each day after school. Diane agreed to engage Sarah in doing tasks in the kitchen while preparing supper. Sarah's son agreed to spend time reminiscing with her while listening to music. This would relieve Diane to enjoy her immediate family in the evening.

I also suggested videos of places Sarah had traveled to with the dance troupe. Perhaps videos of dance would be entertaining, but I warned that they might bring out feelings of loss for Sarah. Her response to each activity would be monitored for adjustment.

The hired helper Sarah liked the majority of the time was described as engaging "in a soft way," slow moving, patient and armed with ideas for bringing Sarah joy. The worker Sarah liked the least was task-oriented, looking for things to do rather than ways to relate.

- People need to feel useful; doing things reduces many negative behaviors. Find activities that are familiar and enjoyable.

- Mood is contagious; a calm care partner often evokes calm in the person being cared for.

- Care partnering is easier if approached with a team effort.

Anecdote—Keep the Lady Moving!

Connie was a very high energy, woman, wiry, restless and pacing the floor. She needed activity that would use up that energy. She didn't recognize the function of an item (this is called agnosia) and would eventually get into unsafe or irritating situations using up some of that energy. She didn't understand the stove would burn, and would often reach over her son Ron while he was cooking to "feel" the boiling stew. We had to find safe things for her to do and help her use up some of her energy and satisfy her curiosity.

I told Ron that long standing over-learned behaviors are retained longest. What had Connie done for a long time? With three children I knew she had probably washed, ironed, cooked, swept, etc. We listed some activities she had found enjoyable and planned to engage her daily. Poisons and cleaners were locked up. Clutter was cleared. Valuables were removed. Important paperwork was hidden. Harmless items like paper plates, plastic containers, pieces of cloth, clothespins and spools of thread were left in view to try to engage her. These familiar visual reminders evoked pleasant memories of days gone by. She spent much time handling them and smiling.

Ron emptied some old clothes from an abandoned bureau upstairs and piled them in a laundry basket. Then he asked her if she'd help him by folding the laundry. She was delighted to help. A mother of three children has done lots of laundry!

After she had folded the clothes, he took the basket upstairs and, depending on her memory loss to assist him in his plan, unfolded and fluffed all the clothes and replaced them in the basket. "Wow, I found some laundry. Can you help me by folding it?" Again she was delighted to help. This ritual continued throughout the day to use up her energy and avoid restlessness and pacing. Sweeping and dry mopping, as well as washing plastic dishes at the sink helped, too.

Ron was the most eager, willing student I've encountered. He made it his business to learn how to work with his mother in a new way. He said he had a new mother and needed to get to know her and what made her happy to be with him. Both he and his mother benefited from his efforts.

- Energy has to be expended in meaningful (to the person) activity that is success oriented. Find meaningful activity for your care partner.

- Depend on long term memory to remain for over-learned behaviors.

- Allow rummaging and pacing as ways to work off energy.

- When energy is not expended, a person may become irritable and possibly aggressive.

- Shadowing is a way to feel active and safe. They are with you!

Anecdote—Redefine What a Meaningful Activity Is

While facilitating a support group of care partners recently, I asked how they adapted their relationships to the memory disorder. One woman talked about her husband doing "weird" things he never would have done before, things that were really bothering her. I asked her to elaborate. It is always good to define words like weird, bizarre or crazy. She explained. "He takes apart the Sunday newspaper pulling the sale flyers out, and then goes through them in detail, underlining things in red." She continued, "He was never interested in shopping. I asked him why he was wasting time looking at the sales inserts. He replied that he was looking for bargains. I said, 'You never wanted to do that before; why now?'"

I asked this woman why she thought it was a waste of time. She reiterated that her husband had never been interested in bargains or shopping. "He used to read the complete paper on Sunday. It disturbs me to see him do this mundane, useless activity. He doesn't read the news anymore. He owned a large business," she continued. "He is so intelligent and capable. It's hard to see him doing little that is productive."

This wife was grieving the loss of the husband she knew, admired and depended on. We talked about the meaning of activity, albeit seemingly wasted time; activity uses up energy that if not expended could turn into restlessness and irritability. The activity used up time doing something orderly and meaningful to him, and avoided his "shadowing" her to find his way into another activity.

"I guess if it is a choice of his hovering about, looking for me to give him something to do, and his scanning the inserts for bargains, I guess I'd better just let it be," she determined.

Being actively involved in what they perceive as purposeful activity, whether it be rummaging, pacing, sorting, separating, stacking items, scanning a newspaper insert or doing a repetitious activity, is a way to find meaning in the day. Sweeping the walk or the garage, washing and/or drying the dishes, packing the washing machine, shoveling and digging holes for planting are all meaningful activities that make a person feel useful. We all get up in the morning because our life today has meaning. But we have a plan. What if you couldn't think of a thing to do that would satisfy your need to have meaning? Perhaps you'd resort to rummaging, sorting, rearranging, stacking, etc. The alternative behavior may be undesirable for all concerned.

Anecdote—The Tower of Babel

Leo had been a mason and enjoyed putting things together. His wife Janet was very sympathetic to Leo's inability to work for a living and turned a blind eye to his seemingly senseless activities at home. Family provided him with brick, stone, cement, wood and nails to keep him engaged in work he was familiar with.

One day Janet came home to find him smiling broadly as he greeted her at the door. He said, "I made you a window box." Leo led her into the living room where he had indeed built her a window box, inside the living room window. He had also paneled the room in odd pieces of wood. She could only accept his "present" and thank him for the good job.

Another time Leo built an outdoor grille for the family with stone and brick. It looked more like a tower of some kind and had no opening for cooking. Again she said it was beautiful. Janet was one of the most compassionate and patient caregivers I've ever met. Leo never felt ridiculed or unappreciated.

- Activity that the person finds satisfying is useful in reducing tension in the mind and body that needs to be expended. It provides meaning to one's day.

- Do not discourage the person from engaging in any safe activity, even if you see no sense in it. Its usefulness is its purposefulness to her.

- Find activity that will expend energy.

- Don't just suggest the activity, set it up. For example, handing a man a broom to sweep the garage is going to be more successful that asking him to sweep the garage but giving him nothing to "remind" him of the request.

Anecdote—Going for an Outing

Rose offered many opportunities for me to try new approaches. She was vehemently independent and needed to feel she was in charge all the time. Her daughter Gloria was stymied over how to get her mother out for an evening meal. If she came to take her mom out dressed with gloves and a hat, Rose would spend many minutes trying to find her own gloves and hat. (She had lost them all.) She would go through each drawer in her apartment looking for the accessories.

This delay happened every time and was very irritating to Gloria. She would tell her mother to hurry up. "You don't need them! We're going in my warm car." They generally would end up arguing. As a result, Rose often refused to go out with her daughter at all.

I suggested that Gloria leave her hat and gloves in the car so Rose wouldn't be visually reminded to want them for herself. Also, I suggested Gloria buy a set of hat and gloves for Rose to be left in the car as well. Gloria had learned that using logic and reasoning often led to argument.

- Visual cues are powerful reminders of past behaviors.

- Logic and reasoning are not effective; the brain cannot them. Avoid these; you will end up arguing.

- Instead of telling your family member to do something, which feels controlling, offer a visual cue that "tells" the mind to respond accordingly.

Anecdote—Use Visual Cues to Avoid Argument

Seventy-year-old Rachel lived with her daughter Angie and her family. Several evenings in a row an argument had begun after dinner between Angie and her mother. Rachel customarily sat at the kitchen table as Angie did the dishes. After sitting at the table a while, Rachel would ask, "Where is my supper? All of you ate and you gave me nothing to eat?"

Angie would try to explain that she had eaten and listed the items she had eaten. Rachel would argue, "No I didn't. Are you trying to starve me or aren't I good enough to eat your food?" In exasperation Angie would give in and prepare another plate for her mother. This wasn't a good idea as Rachel had diabetes and shouldn't have eaten two meals.

······· *Pause for thought* ·····························

What would you suggest Angie do?

_____

_____

_____

_____

_____

With memory loss, people often need something visual to let them know what is or has happened. I suggested that Angie leave her mother's dirty plate and silverware, and perhaps a full glass of water or cup of tea on the table to occupy her while Angie did the supper dishes. She was then instructed to invite her mother to bring over her dishes and wash them. By leaving the dirty plate before her, Rachel was "re-minded" that she had eaten. It avoided argument and Rachel's feeling her needs were being disregarded. Then, after Rachel washed her dish, both were to immediately retreat to the living room to join the rest of the family, thus eliminating the visual cue of the meal site.

- Memory loss creates a false sense of what has just happened.

- A visual cue will "remind" the brain, and eliminate confusion and possibly an argument!

- Use visual cues, or the removal of one, to change behavior.

Anecdote—I Didn't Order That!

This same visual cueing approach worked in a slightly different way for staff at a local assisted living residence. I was doing a training session with the staff. A wait staff person told about a resident who asked for one meal choice but when it was brought to her complained, "I didn't order that. I want the other choice, what she has," pointing to her table companion. Another meal was brought to her only to have her say she hadn't ordered that and wanted the first choice! What to do?

I suggested to the staff member that this woman probably had immediate memory loss and wasn't simply being cantankerous. She had no history of being difficult about other services provided.

"She had no memory of ordering the first meal when it came," I explained, "and the visual cue of the meal her table companion had was inviting." If they brought her a second choice, I suggested leaving the first one there for a while to "remind" her she had ordered both. If she started eating after a few minutes, they were not to bring the second choice. If she still insisted she didn't want the first choice, they were to bring the second and leave both on the table. Since there was no third choice, she had two options and either one would be all right with the staff. Sometimes she ate both! Either way, a meal would have had to be wasted.

- Satisfy the need for choice using visual cues

- Keep the mood neutral or positive when confronted by negative behavior.

- Do not assume bothersome behavior is intentionally to irritate. Think outside the box! It may be the best the person can do without immediate memory.

Anecdote—Visual Cues Encourage Independence

Hazel was eighty-nine and enjoyed working part time at a local department store curtain department. She had suffered many illnesses herself and was determined to stay active. Henry, her husband, had Alzheimer's disease. Hazel wondered if she could still maintain her work schedule and care for him, too. Henry was mobile, took walks without any episodes of getting lost and could keep himself busy safely for the few hours she was gone.

Remembering to eat lunch, however, was a challenge for Henry. When Hazel returned home, he complained about being hungry. He had lost his ability to organize a small meal independently. Hazel was aware of his short term memory loss.

Together we devised a system to help Henry to eat lunch. We set up a clock on the kitchen table set to sound an alarm at noon, his usual lunch time. In front of the clock a place mat, glass and silverware were set up. We hoped the place setting would prompt Henry to read the card on the plate which said,

HENRY'S LUNCH IN FRIDGE

Would this prompt him to go to the fridge? On the door of the fridge was a second sign. It read,

HENRY'S LUNCH INSIDE

Not leaving anything to chance, on top of his lunch we placed a sign reading,

HENRY'S LUNCH

This cueing worked for several months and Hazel happily continued working 10-1:30. Obviously this could only work if Henry was able to understand words. Some with dementia lose this ability early in the disease process.

- Use consistent, familiar visual cues to help a person with dementia perform everyday tasks. It will give him a feeling of self confidence and purpose.

- It is much better to set up a task to be successful than take over a task for her.

Anecdote—Use Visual Cueing to Stop Unwanted Behaviors

Fanny is eighty-two and lives with her daughter Sue, who complained that during toileting, her mother would pick at the disposable protective underwear. She would continue until it was in shreds and unable to be used, although clean. This was not only annoying to Sue, but becoming expensive. Sue began dreading the toileting scene! No amount of reprimand seemed to work. In fact, the reprimands had led to her mother weeping. Sue admitted she was often exasperated even before she toileted Fanny. If Sue tried to stop Fanny from picking at the underwear, Fanny would try to raise herself off the toilet to end the conflict. Sue was worried about her falling and wanted Fanny to sit long enough to finish toileting.

Pause for thought

What would you do to stop behavior that is annoying and wasteful?

_____

_____

_____

_____

_____

Upon questioning Sue, I learned that Fanny took twenty to thirty minutes or longer to toilet. I guessed that as she became restless sitting so long, the underwear became a focus to ease her restlessness. She needed something to keep her hands busy; the underwear was the only object that was visible (remember the power of visual cues) and readily available. Although not a useful activity, it was satisfying her need to do something.

I suggested that Sue cover Fanny's legs to above the underwear with a towel, and give her something to hold or manipulate that would keep her interest. Sue recalled her mother's fascination with bright fabrics and yarns. We decided to sew ribbons, large buttons and various other familiar and attractive items onto the towel so it became her focus for busyness rather than the paper underwear. The "busy apron" was secured around Fanny's waist with a broad bright colored ribbon. She was able to sit for the half hour and keep busy with something enjoyable rather than busying herself picking apart the costly protective underwear, and she no longer tried to raise herself off the toilet. Seeing her mother content to sit and fiddle, Sue could now approach the task without the anticipation of another unpleasant time together.

- Replace activity that is unhelpful, wasteful or annoying with something else to do that brings pleasure.

- Avoid reprimand; it is not helpful.

Anecdote -Our mother with a doll? Never!

I was coaching two sisters in the care of their mother. When they talked of her restless wandering about the house, following them around, I suggested a baby doll or stuffed animal as a way of engaging her in an activity she knew well: that of caring for someone. They both exclaimed in unison, "Our mom would never be seen holding a stuffed toy!" I convinced them to try. Next visit I brought a stuffed bear and asked their mother to mind it while I talked with her daughters. She said she would. She proceeded to the sofa and, talking softly to the bear began rocking gently back and forth. She was contented for an hour. When I left, I said I'd leave the bear with her to care for. She was delighted, walking off down the hall, carrying the bear. The daughters were very surprised. They had been unable to accept that the needs of their mother had changed due to her illness. She needed something to care for. The bear was now her "baby."

Toward the end of the disease when activity the person can participate actively in is past, it is possible to offer stimulation of a passive nature. Remember that emotional memory is not affected in dementia, so throughout the disease we can offer pleasurable pastimes. Objects that appeal to the senses are helpful, such as a soft stuffed animal to hold, things to manipulate and things to look at, smell or taste.

Anecdote- A trip back in time to WW II

Bernard was completely bedridden, needing to be moved with a Hoyer lift. He could not hold up his weight and sat in a wheelchair when up. His wife, determined to care for him at home until his death, was looking for ways to keep him happy. I found out he had been an Air Force pilot in WW II and adored planes. We found a mobile of planes that, when a breeze came in the window, gently rotated. Bernard found much pleasure in these planes, often talking to them about wartime.

When he was up in the wheelchair, to avoid restlessness we purchased a large, busy box of rotating wheels, cranks and sliding levers, and secured it to a tray attached to the wheelchair. Bernard busied himself with manipulating the various items over and over. It is hard for a family to think of an adult enjoying such simple pleasures; they think it is childish. It is child-like, but that was the level of functioning Bernie had at the time. His wife was surprised at his response and kept thinking of other simple things to keep him entertained.

Anecdote -Old interests still entertain

Tapping into old interests helped George's wife Lucille, who had been his first mate for years on their thirty-three-foot sailboat. George knew something had changed cognitively when, one day, while standing at the bow to pick up the anchor, she froze in that standing position with no idea how to proceed. When I met them, Lucille was confined to an easy chair and had no speech. George and I talked about what her interests were besides sailing. I discovered she had loved doing puzzles like Rubik Cubes, interlaced chains, etc. I asked if he still had some of these puzzles. Yes, he said, they were in the attic.

We placed an over-bed table in front of the chair where Lucille sat and put one or two of these puzzles in front of her. On a table nearby we set up a music box to play water music they used to listen to while sailing. George was content when he saw Lucille's pleasure in these objects.

- Emotional response is present to the end of a dementia-causing disease.

- Use objects that are reminders of activities that were enjoyed when the person was well.

- Passive participation in activities is still engaging him in something.

- Objects that appeal to the senses (seeing, hearing, smelling, tasting, feeling) are good for people in the end stage of a dementing illness.

Challenge #6:

SAFETY

Providing safety is sometimes a challenge. People want to continue habits and activities that brought them satisfaction in the past. This may be shopping, going to church, cooking, etc. But some of these activities can become a safety concern. Is the person safe at the stove? Can the person manage money, buy with discrimination? Is she able to find her way safely to a destination? All these questions must be assessed on an ongoing basis and, when needed, an intervention must be developed to ensure safety.

Anecdote—Marie's Own Shrine

Marie's mom lives at a rest home, which is not secure (locked). She does well for the most part, with help, with hygiene and socialization. But a safety concern arose; Marie's mom had always gone to her church each morning to pray. She continued this practice at the church on the same street as the rest home. Marie worried about her mom's mobility and hearing deficits, which made her trip to church risky. Marie also worried about her mom's judgment crossing that street, yet she didn't want to deprive her of her daily ritual.

Pause for thought

Would you discourage her from going to church to pray?

_____

_____

_____

_____

Perhaps, I suggested, she would be satisfied if the church came to her. Maybe a place of her own where she could pray for her family and friends would help. Marie's mom needed a sacred place to say her prayers.

Marie approached the local church for ideas. The church donated a small statue to the rest home and the maintenance crew at the rest home erected it in the yard just outside her room. Surrounded with plantings and a bench, it became her personal shrine. Marie suggested to her mother that she could now pray for her friends and other concerns many times daily at her own shrine. She promised to take her mother to church on Sunday as usual and perhaps one additional day.

Presented in a helpful light, her mom became enamored with her own personal place of worship. News of her shrine reached other residents in the rest home, who admired it and shared in her joy. Marie goes to this special place throughout the day, which prevents the need to walk to church.

- Offer acceptable substitutes in situations that present safety concerns.

- No meaningful activity should be denied the person with dementia if at all possible.

Anecdote—Making Bathing Safe

Connie's bathing was a challenge. Connie is the wiry high energy lady we talked about earlier, remember? Not always recognizing Ron as her son, she would refuse his assistance bathing. After many attempts to explain why she needed to bathe, he gave up trying to get her in the upstairs shower and sponge bathed her downstairs in the kitchen. The shower stall upstairs was small and the bathroom was dark and up a steep flight of stairs. I didn't think it was an inviting place either;

I agreed with Connie's reluctance to go there with a "stranger" who wanted to bathe her!

Terry, a home care aide, helped Ron bathe his mother each day, but Connie put up quite a fight. When Terry attempted to remove her protective underwear, Connie would grab Terry's wrists in fear, digging her nails into her. Terry had sustained deep scratches and didn't know what to do.

Pause for thought

Can you devise a plan to help protect Terry from harm and bath Connie?

_____

_____

_____

_____

_____

Together, Ron, Terry and I devised a possible solution. Aware a person with dementia finds it extremely difficult, if not impossible, to attend to two things at the same time, we gave her a large towel and kept repeating, "Hold it tight, Connie. You don't want anyone to see!" Connie also couldn't distinguish that the television programming was not happening in the room and would talk to the people on TV. We placed a towel over the television screen while bathing her, as she thought the news anchor could see her. She liked his voice but didn't want him staring at her!

Wrapping the towel around her while she was still dressed and giving the ends to her to hold on to, Terry, humming softly, stood in front of Connie (the visual cue), repeating for her to hold the towel close to her while she proceeded to wash Connie's body. Ron removed the soiled underwear from behind, avoiding the necessity of Terry bending and being out of Connie's eyeshot. Ron standing behind out of her sight prevented the visual cueing of two persons. "Don't drop the towel, Connie. Hold on tight." Terry repeated whenever it appeared Connie was distracted from her task. Once she was washed, Connie willingly allowed clean, dry underwear and clothing to be put on.

Later on in the disease, when Ron washing her was not unpleasant or frightening anymore, and during the summer months when it was hot, Ron placed a sturdy plastic chair in a child's yard pool, which he set in the front foyer. He poured warm water from a kettle over Connie's lower body while she, sitting, as before, held the towel around her upper body. This way she received a "shower." After the shower, Ron pulled the pool to the front door and folded it to allow the water to cascade down the front stairs. "I kill two birds with one stone," he said. "I clean my mother and the front stairs."

Ron would try anything even if it seemed ludicrous, and thought up a few innovative strategies of his own. Both Ron and Connie are deceased now but not forgotten. I learned a great deal being his coach.

- There is more than one way to get clean!

- You sometimes have to develop a care partnering team.

- Always preserve the person's dignity when performing personal tasks like bathing and toileting.

Anecdote—Minimize Agitation to Stay Safe

Jack was becoming more irritable during mornings, making his small-framed wife afraid he would become physically aggressive. Jack was a large man, a military retiree and a former law enforcement officer. He was frequently asking, "What do I do now?" when attempting simple tasks of daily living. Sequencing skills were diminishing rapidly. He was depending on Lois for step by step instruction.

Jack's agitation escalated when Lois told him it was time to bathe. He resisted and yelled at her, "I don't want to!" She persisted in urging him so he would get to the day program on time. Their son was also fearful his mom would be hurt if she pushed him to do things. "Maybe he doesn't want to bathe first," he suggested. "Why not let him eat breakfast first, Mom?"

Perhaps Jack was hungry when he woke, leading to the irritability. He had developed type 2 diabetes, which may have contributed to his need for food and to his irritability. I suggested that beginning the day with a task that was becoming more difficult for Jack to perform was cause for his agitation. So Lois agreed to try reversing the tasks. Jack sat at the table while Lois made breakfast, acclimating himself to the new day. He was much more agreeable to bathing after a good breakfast!

- Adjust the schedule to do the familiar and desired task first.

- People need choices to enhance self efficacy.

- People are often disoriented upon awakening. Work slowly, giving yourself time so you are not feeling rushed.

Anecdote—Minimize Aggressive Behavior If You Can't Eliminate It

Victoria and Vincent had been married for forty-five years. Vincent describes his wife as having been an "angel of a woman," hard working and accomplished. She had worked up to a position in management at a large company. Since being diagnosed with Alzheimer's disease, she had become increasingly aggressive verbally and lately physically as well. Vincent was not a well man, having suffered a heart attack necessitating open heart surgery. Victoria kicked, hit and bit him under paranoid and delusional thinking. The situation was unsafe for both Victoria and Vincent.

On her healthier side, she was able to easily bathe, dress appropriately, groom, telephone family and friends and complete some housekeeping. She was articulate and presented well to neighbors, friends and some family. Others had a hard time believing Vincent's reports of her abusive behavior.

He said she had accused him of having an affair. He had tried to correct her false belief, defending himself against her additional accusations of his stealing from her, and tried to reason with her. These attempts always led to more aggressive behavior and sometimes she left the house in a rage.

Vincent was very discouraged and feeling powerless to work with his wife, but he wanted to care for her at home. He worried that when she ran from home enraged she'd get lost, but he didn't know what to do.

I taught him that he couldn't use logic and reasoning any more and that her paranoid delusions about infidelity were "fixed"; he would not be able to explain them away. I suggested that he find a pleasurable activity to use up some of her pent up energy. Her inactivity led to irritability and subsequent aggressive behavior.

We looked at the triggers for her behavior and decided to remove the triggers as much as possible. They were talk of, or visual reminders of, her money, jewelry and mail. Worry about their disappearing evoked anxiety for Victoria.

I encouraged Vincent to invite her to help him make meals and clean up after so she felt engaged in something meaningful and familiar. I also strongly advised him to avoid argument and the use of logic. I asked him to apologize (even if he wasn't wrong) to help her calm down if she showed anger. Perhaps, I thought, engaging in familiar tasks with her husband would present him in a more benevolent light and the aggression against him would stop.

I also felt it unsafe and unkind to allow her to suffer the psychotic symptoms and agitation. It is very frightening to be psychotic and it is emotionally painful to be agitated. Medication to alleviate her fears and unreal thinking was sought. An adult day program to give her structure was suggested, gaining her cooperation by saying it was a volunteer position. This is, again, a fiblet used for her benefit. Victoria was known to pride herself on her helpfulness to others in need. As she had no idea that she needed structure in her day, presenting the day program to her, as a way of helping others might make it palatable.

- Point out positive behaviors; avoid criticizing the negative ones.

- Avoid the use of logic and reasoning.

- Delusional and paranoid ideation cannot be explained away. If it evokes dangerous behavior, medication may be needed.

- Choose activity that is familiar and meaningful to the person

- Mood is contagious; calm creates calm, anger, more anger.

- Antipsychotic medications are only used when the delusion is disturbing. If it is a pleasant delusion for the person, let it be. Enter their reality and enjoy it with them.

An aside about asking the doctor for medications:

Some doctors seem averse to prescribing antipsychotic medication (medication to ease delusions and hallucinations leading to aggressive or other unsafe behaviors). If they feel the request is to free up the family, the physician may be hesitant and medication may be denied. I suggest that the family talk about the patient's great distress and ask for relief for her. Your family member needs an advocate in her treatment.

Anecdote—Understand What Triggers Aggression

Frank was severely impaired cognitively but very mobile. He would pace and rummage; a safety problem existed because he didn't recognize the use of objects. He would pick up an object and, not knowing what it was for, use it unsafely. His wife Sue had put away everything that she felt could be used improperly.

One morning, upon entering the kitchen, she saw Frank just about to drink liquid dish detergent. It was yellow, just about the color of lemonade. She had learned that he could react defensively out of fear if she yelled to stop or pulled the detergent out of his hand. She was afraid he'd strike her, which he had done once before. Instead she bumped up against him, flipping the bottle of detergent out of his hand, to the floor.

"Oh, how clumsy I am! I'm sorry, Frank. Let me get you something else to drink." She quickly took out orange juice from the refrigerator and poured him a glass. He said, "Its okay. This drink is very good and tasty. Thank you."

How differently this could have been had Sue reacted instead of responded. She had learned not to react. Frank might have hurt her or he might have lost his balance and fallen. An argument might have followed, resulting in Sue feeling badly and Frank confused and upset about what the argument was about. (By the way, he would have won the argument!) Unable to process argument, he would have repeated one phrase such as "I don't understand why you pick on me," or, "I didn't do anything wrong; leave me alone," or, "Give that back to me right now!"

• Try not to alarm a person with dementia; they will do something to express this alarm. It could be unsafe for them or for you!

• Remove any liquid or object in the home that could be used unsafely by your family member with memory loss.

• Learn to think a minute before you respond to a behavior that is potentially harmful.

People with dementia can become agitated and perhaps subsequently hurtful to their care partners. Learning what can cause agitation is very important in preventing unwanted behaviors that are a result of fear or loss of dignity.

The following are some causes of agitation:

1. Being in his personal space (during bathing or dressing, toileting) can cause aggressive behavior. An acceptable space between us and a stranger is arm's length. This is not possible during the above tasks of hygiene and grooming, especially if the recipient doesn't remember who you are. As he learns to trust you, he may accept, even welcome being physically closer.

2. Frustration from being asked to do something she cannot do anymore (tie a shoe, dress, bathe, make a sandwich) can lead to agitation. If she is historically easily frustrated, this may be a frequent response. You must learn low-frustration

approaches to reduce the likeliness of her acting out her aggravation.

3. Being asked an open-ended question—what, when, how, who, why—can result in irritability. Open-ended questions are too hard to process, therefore too hard to answer. He may simply not answer or become irritated. Reframe the question to be answered yes or no, or choose between no more than two choices.4. For example, instead of asking, "What did you do today?" ask, "Did you have a good day today?" Because it is an easier question to process, he may even recall something that made it a good day. Never ask, "Why did you do that?" or "Why are you angry?" He doesn't know. He can't tell you. Instead, say, "You just _____(e.g. pounded the table). Did something upset you?" Now he may be able to answer the question.

4. Inability to tell others what she wants to say can lead to frustration and evoke a negative response. (Try talking to someone whose language is different from yours and see how tired you get.)

5. If he sees no logic in doing something you ask him to do, he may respond unfavorably. This often happens when you urge him to bathe and he doesn't see why he should.

6. She may not understand what we expect of her. For example, offering an activity that she cannot easily perform anymore and expecting her to do it is confusing to him. We need to observant of her present abilities and adjust our expectations accordingly.

7. He may be responding to a loss of dignity, lack of choice or loss of control of his life (this may be real or perceived).

8. Inactivity or not enough to do builds restlessness in the body. She may respond to this restlessness by becoming irritable.

9. Discomfort (pain, hunger, thirst) he cannot tell you about or that you are unaware of can cause aggression. It is like when a pre-verbal child slaps his hand on your arm to get your attention. This could be perceived as aggression, except that the child is three feet tall, not six feet.

10. Lack of sleep (this makes us all a bit irritable) can cause agitation.

11. Medication side effects (therapeutic or toxic doses) are another cause for negative behaviors. Elders are sensitive to drugs anyway and can become toxic easily. If a drug is started at too high a dose, increased too rapidly or not taken correctly, the side effect can be agitated behavior. Some medications that are given for aggression can cause it in certain people and in certain dementia causing illnesses.

12. Agitation can be a response to our stress or speaking to her in an unsupportive way (disrespectful, demeaning, bossy).

13. Negative response to touch can cause irritability; some persons with dementia love to be touched; others don't and try to "brush you away." This can be viewed as aggressiveness.

14. Feeling isolated, insecure or frightened can lead to her "telling someone" by hitting them. In a film called The Great Brain Robbery by Joanne Koenig Coste, one patient says, "I can't whisper anymore, I can only scream!"

When the cause for alarm is not corrected or the emotional need is not satisfied, agitation may escalate to aggressive behavior. Examine negative behavior for its meaning. (Refer back to the discussion on behavior and its meaning).

Challenge #7:
CARE PARTNER STRESS

When care partners talk about the behaviors that stress them the most, each person's vulnerability or level of tolerance is different. What bothers one person minimally can be a real problem for another. Some behaviors that seemed to be most bothersome to care partners are repeated questioning, shadowing, wandering and the desire to "go home." Others found lack of cooperation a real challenge, and for others the lack of communication was most missed. It is a good practice to list those behaviors that bother you the most and work on understanding them. Find new responses to them that will bring about a new behavior.

Pause for thought

List some behaviors of your family member you find most frustrating. Develop some new ways to respond to those behaviors based on what you have learned thus far.

_____

_____

_____

_____

_____

_____

_____

Learning the use of fiblets is invaluable in handling some of these behaviors, thereby reducing your stress. Let's talk some more about fiblets.

Fiblets Gain Cooperation

Fiblets are little untruths in the service of the person with dementia. The rationale in using fiblets is that they help gain cooperation, they keep the person (or the care partner) safe, they preserve the person's dignity, they help neutralize a toxic situation and they satisfy an immediate emotional need.

Anecdote—Appeal to the Need for Control by Using Fiblets
A problem arose for Ted and the staff where his mother Grace lived. Grace wouldn't go to dinner in the assisted living residence until "her family" arrived. There were two seatings for meals in the residence, and the last one was over by seven p.m. Grace also insisted that she would not be subjected to adhering by a specific time to eat and that she would "dine tonight at eight o'clock"! Grace would appear at eight to an empty dining room and demand something to eat from the dining room staff cleaning up the kitchen. Unfortunately, trying to accommodate her, they reinforced this habit.

Learning that Grace was an only child who all through life had gotten her way, I suggested a different approach, counting on her immediate memory loss to help make the approach work. I instructed the resident care aide to say at mealtime, "Grace, everyone is waiting for you in the dining room. No one will start to eat until you arrive."

Grace would quickly pat her nose with powder, put on fresh lipstick and go with the aide readily. This worked because she had no memory of the conversation that preceded her going to the dining room; when she got there she made no comment that no one acknowledged her arrival and that they were happily engaged in dining.

She was given control by appealing to her ego. Everyone was indeed already eating and, because she had no memory of what she had been told upstairs, she could be led to her usual place at a table for four without incident. This approach worked for five years, three times daily. She never did give up her need for her own way!

- Use approaches that consider the personality and validation of her value.

- Your stress can be alleviated by thinking outside the box for solutions to uncooperative behaviors.

Anecdote—Use Fiblets to Save a Person's Dignity

Fay's husband Frank wanted to drive her places. She felt quite uneasy about his driving, but whenever she offered an alternative plan for getting places he got angry, which was unlike him. Fay didn't want him to drive, but when she tried to explain why he shouldn't drive, it led to argument every time. (Explaining often does!) Frank had no memory of his doctor telling him to stop driving and he believed he drove well, so Fay's reasoning with him often led to not going at all. Fay was feeling powerless. She continued to let him drive her.

One day Frank told her he was going to the store for three or four items. She suggested he write a list.

"No, I'll remember the items," Frank countered. When she insisted he write it down, he said, "You write the list."

"No, you write the list. You've always complained about not being able to read my writing anyway," she reasoned.

This led to an argument about who would write the list. Fay wondered what prompted him to get so upset. I suggested that perhaps he couldn't easily write and was avoiding doing so.

She wanted to see if he could write a list and follow it. If he was having trouble writing, this was a recent change in his cognitive status and it scared her. This meant the disease was progressing.

I had met Fay at a support group. I spoke that day about preserving relationship, avoiding argument, eliminating long explanations and the use of fiblets to preserve dignity and control. Later she reported the following to me. "I had a doctor's appointment and didn't want him driving me, but I didn't want another argument either." Using her new knowledge of fiblets, she informed Frank that she'd asked their daughter to take her to her appointment with the doctor for a test. She quickly added, "There will be several forms to be filled out while I'm having the test."

Frank had never acknowledged his difficulty writing, but, when told there'd be forms to fill out, he seemed relieved that someone else taking her for her appointment. This use of a fiblet (there actually were no forms to sign) saved face for Frank, relieved Fay of an anxious trip to the doctor as a passenger, and avoided another argument that would have ended with both losing!

- It is important to keep the person with dementia from being embarrassed.

- Telling him that he can't do something when he has no awareness of his inability to do it safely only points out his failings and leads to having bad feelings about his care partner.

- Create a positive experience for the person with dementia, even if you have to tell fiblets. That is what they are for!

- Taking away driving privilege is a major hurdle for most people.

Anecdote—Use Fiblets to Address the Need to "Go Home"

Leo resides at an assisted living residence where he can be kept safe from harm. He had been leaving his home and threatening his wife if she tried to stop him. He was found a few times by family and once luckily by the local police department as he walked along a busy highway.

His wife Iris, however, was sad about his being away from home and felt guilty that she had brought him there. Her children, worried about her health, persuaded her that the move was in everyone's best interest.

Iris wept as she told me how Leo pleads with her each time she ends her visit with him, "Why are you leaving without me? Why can't I come with you?" She would cry all the way home and was struggling with her indecision about whether to leave him at the assisted living or take him home.

I reminded her that he had asked to go home when he was home. She told me he'd insist, "I know this is my furniture and you're Iris, but this is not my home. I have to go home. Take me now!" When Iris refused or tried to explain that he was home, he became angry. This would lead to him leaving for one of his exploratory walks to find "home."

I encouraged her in the decision to allow him to remain at the assisted living and helped her reduce her stress when the visit ended. "Tell him you'll be right back and make a reason for leaving the immediate area. For example, you need to confer with a person out in the hall outside the locked doors or you have to use the ladies room." I instructed her not to kiss him goodbye as this would signal that her visit was over.

Home is the place where we feel safe and at ease. When a person with memory loss and confusion asks for home, he often is expressing a feeling of confusion and lack of emotional safety. Responding to that need is more helpful than "explaining" why he cannot go home.

Iris needed to know that she represented safety and clarity to Leo wherever they were at the moment, and when she left it meant his "home" was going, too. I advised her not to take him away from the residence for several weeks, and then to go someplace besides their home. I also suggested that she take along another person, preferably a male, to help her if Leo resisted returning.

Moving a spouse to another home is wrought with emotion. Guilty feelings that she was abandoning Leo or giving up on him made ending her visits with Leo difficult for Iris. Since the rest of the visit usually went very well, filled with conversation, enjoying music together and reminiscing, it was obvious that it was Iris' leaving that was traumatic. She saved Leo that separation anxiety by not being entirely honest with him.

- Home is a descriptive word to express comfort and safety.

Anecdote—Use Fiblets to Distract

Monica's father waited at the door of their apartment building, dressed in outdoor wear. He told her he was waiting for his brother, who he said had called to have dinner out with them. Knowing her uncle had died many years ago, Monica told her father that perhaps his brother's plane was late. "Why don't you come to dinner and reception will tell him we are there?"

This did not satisfy her father. He continued to stand firm. "I'll wait for him here like I said I would. Leave me here. You go eat."

138

No amount of "explaining" or persuading budged him. He became irritable, but thanks to his social manners didn't lose his temper in the building's reception area. After an hour of persisting, Monica was able to convince her father to join them in the dining area. She was exhausted and didn't enjoy the meal at all. Nothing had been accomplished.

She called me to get coaching in this matter. I wondered if her father might have responded better to being told his brother had called to tell Monica he was being delayed and that they should start dinner. I suggested she say, "He didn't want you waiting so he called and wants to meet us in the dining room for dessert."

Knowing why his brother might be late was not enough to satisfy her father's need to be waiting for his brother. In addition, she was reasoning with her father without finding a way to satisfy his need. Being a controlling, opinionated man, he wasn't ready to concede to what Monica thought. He wanted to know what his brother's desires were and have dessert ready for him when he arrived.

- Fiblets are used to satisfy the immediate emotional need.

- When using fiblets to change behavior, think what need the person is expressing by the behavior. It may be the need for promptness or politeness to another, like in this case, or a need to be included in plans. Discover what will satisfy the person's need and supply it with a fiblet.

Anecdote—Use Fiblets to Gain Connection and Trust, and to Enter Their Reality

I visited a client's husband at her request to see whether I thought he could adjust to living away from her in the assisted living residence where he had been for two weeks. Nicole was finding caring for him at home emotionally draining. She hadn't been sleeping, fearful he would leave the home during the night. She also didn't believe she could tolerate coordinating hired, in-home helpers. "I can't orchestrate that and I can't do it all myself," she explained. But she felt guilty about this and wanted an outside person's opinion about the wisdom of her decision.

I wasn't sure how aware Jim was of where he was and asked staff about what they were doing to keep him engaged with them. "We tell him he is helping us learn how to run the place. He was in charge of setting up businesses in his work life. He tells us he'll stay just three more days, and if we can't get it right by then, he is leaving the assignment."

I asked what happened after three days. "He isn't aware time has passed, so he tells us each day he'll try to help us organize ourselves for only three more days."

With this information I approached him. "Hi, I'm Beverly. I was sent to find out how you're getting on with this business here." Jim never asked me who sent me or who I was. He looked very relaxed and whispered, "I don't know if they'll ever get organized. They don't seem to understand."

"Is this a hotel?" I asked.

"I guess something like a hotel. The door to my room is locked."

"Oh, so you're staying overnight here, too."

"I think it'll take a few weeks to get them so they're okay without me."

It was apparent he was feeling useful and that the staff had helped him in that regard. He had been entering into activities, too, which indicated his comfort level. When I told him I had to leave and thanked him for his report, he escorted me to the locked door, called a staff member to open it for me and made no attempt to follow me. He just waved goodbye. I was happy to report back to Nicole that he was adjusting well there; feeling useful and showing no sign of wanting to leave.

- Enter the person's reality and enjoy them there.

- Helping a person feel valued is very important to gaining connection.

- Behavior tells us how a person feels; get away from your feelings for a moment (guilt, grief, fear) and watch what his behavior is 'saying' he is feeling.

Anecdote—Shadowing the Caregiver

Shadowing refers to the person with dementia following or staying close to the care partner. Shadowing is generally fear based; the confused, disoriented or fearful person may only feel safe when the care partner is in sight, or less than a foot away! It is only then that he can he feel grounded in safety. Shadowing is sometimes a lack of the person's ability to initiate an activity that satisfies, so he "attaches" to the care partner for structure and direction.

This is a very annoying behavior to some care partners. Sometimes they feel better when they understand the behavior is fear based. If the shadowing is about a need for structure and direction, it is easier to manage. Provide the person with something meaningful (again, meaningful to him) to do.

Anecdote-A behavior's intent can be puzzling.

Jody and her mom have lived together after the death of Jody's dad. Her mom shadowed her everywhere, even knocking on the door of the bathroom when Jody tried to get some space there. The strain of grieving the loss of her dad and managing her mom was building. Jody came home from a job she disliked to a home that reminded her of her grief and where she was followed until her mother retired at nine o'clock.

I visited Jody and her mom in their home, noting Jody's affect to be sad and her voice flat. She arrived home with many bitter complaints about work and about her coworkers. From time to time her mother would say to Jody, "I'm not a bother, am I? Am I doing something wrong?" Jody would respond in a flat but crisp tone, "No, of course not, why do you ask that?"

I wondered what the shadowing was "saying." (All behavior has meaning!) I suggested to Jody that her mother might be responding to the sadness she felt in her daughter and that perhaps the shadowing was worry about Jody and an attempt to cheer her.

I suggested she do a bit of acting when she came home at night. She was to try to rid herself of the workplace on the way home (perhaps listen to some soothing music and take deep breaths). She was to say upon entering the home, "Boy I'm glad to be home with you. The traffic was wild." She was to smile and give her mother a hug and move slowly about the kitchen while preparing supper. Perhaps continuing the music at home would help Jody stay relaxed as well.

I also suggested she seek counseling for the grief she was unable to talk about with her mother concerning her father's death. Her mother had little memory of her husband at this time.

Jody wasn't able to sustain this approach, so we never found out whether the shadowing was an expression of concern; but I believe it was. While I was talking lightheartedly and Jody seemed to be enjoying herself, her mother had left us to go to the yard and tend to her flowers. As long as the easy conversation continued, Jody's mother was able to leave her daughter and pursue other activity.

- Shadowing may have several causes.

- Affect is contagious.

- Behavior is an expression of a need, a want or a feeling. Explore the possibilities before coming to any conclusion

An important aside: Caring for you lessens your stress.

Care partner stress is real and needs to be tended to. I read somewhere that the stress a caregiver for someone with dementia experiences is like that of a soldier in combat. You, like the soldier, are hyper vigilant, not knowing where the enemy will appear or perhaps even who the enemy is, and usually lacking sufficient sleep to reason it all out. You remain constantly "on call." Many caregivers have said they don't close their eyes at night for long before they have a sense of something about to happen. Some have used baby monitors to help with this uneasiness. Taking care of safety hazards reduces worry.

Support groups, chat lines and a personal coach or counselor can all be very valuable to reduce stress. Support groups can be located at your local state Alzheimer's Association website. You must take care of yourself to be able to care for someone else.

Suggestions for Caring for You

- Pay attention to your needs for socialization and pleasurable activities. Taking care of yourself gives you the reserve to continue to give care with a willing spirit.

- Attend a support group regularly. Learn from others' experiences.

- Continue to learn about the memory disorder your care partner has.

- Ask for help and accept help when it is offered, even if it is a small thing. If you refuse, the help may not be offered again.

- Inform family members about the plan for care, even if they don't seem interested, so there is less chance of disagreement later.

- If there is conflict in the family around caregiving issues, find a family mediator and come to a decision all can accept. Often old issues of conflict arise during a crisis and you will need an outside person to help you deal with it.

- Make sure all legal, financial and health related papers are complete and available: health care proxy, durable power of attorney, etc.

- Elder law firms are expanding their services and can help with planning care, protecting assets and coordinating services with other helpful people and agencies. Elder law attorneys are focused entirely on elder issues and are more apt to stay abreast of new laws.

- Geriatric care managers can help, too, by coordinating services, finding local resources and accessing them for you. You can find out about them from your local elder care agency or online. Google in geriatric care managers or go to www.caremanagers.org.

- Do not expect yourself to always feel good about what you are doing. Caring for someone you love with memory loss is a complex job that changes from day to day. You may find yourself feeling all kinds of emotion, good and bad. Feelings are feelings. It is the behavior that results from the feeling that is important.

• Let the local police department know of your care partner's memory loss and provide them with a recent photograph.

• A Safe Return bracelet from the Alzheimer's Association (1-888-572-8566) helps protect against your care partner being lost. It is a worldwide program that identifies the person with memory loss through an SR number that corresponds to one on a central computer. When accessed, a person, usually a police officer, can identify the person, his next of kin, his home address and many other helpful facts. This is a good safety device to have for the person who no longer knows where he lives or who his family is.

• Many communities in Massachusetts have a program called Project Lifesaver usually connected to the police department or sheriff's office. Ask about it in your state or community. Project Lifesaver in Massachusetts is reportedly successful in finding a person who has wandered away one hundred percent of the time within thirty minutes. It is accomplished through a honing device in a bracelet.

• Turn off the stove when you are not in attendance. Often people will use the stove for unsafe things, like lighting a cigarette, or forget they haven't used a stove in perhaps years. This activity is often the result of lack of supervision and a need to have something to do. You can remove the knobs when you are not in attendance and store them in an unusual place (perhaps the freezer). This will give you peace of mind.

• Make keys inaccessible. People who haven't driven for years may forget this fact and take the keys to the car and take a drive!

Challenge #8:

SEXUALITY

Sexuality is a given. Persons don't cease to be male and female when diagnosed with dementia. Their sexuality may be expressed differently, however. If social appropriateness is lacking due to frontal lobe damage, a person may be quite uninhibited about staying clothed or satisfying the sexual urge.

It is important to acknowledge that each person is a sexual being, and needs affirmation of that in some way. To address an unwanted behavior, direct away from it.

Anecdote-Hold this for me, Charles.

Charles was bathed three times a week by a homecare aide, Louise. She was having concerns about his behavior and his safety. When she washed him, he reached out and grabbed her breasts or buttocks, whatever was within his reach. When she tried to avoid his grasp or tell him to stop, he'd become irate, irritated with her and unsteady on his feet, which then presented a safety problem.

Pause for thought

If you were Louise, what would you do to get Charles to stop grabbing?

_____

_____

_____

_____

Knowing the person with dementia cannot do two things at once, I suggested Louise engage him in "helping" her bathe him. I instructed her to give him a washcloth and soap and to keep telling him to soap up the cloth real good. While he was engaged in that she bathed his body. She hummed to herself to mirror calm, and at the end asked him to wash his private parts. Rinsing him, she'd tell him to put the face-cloth under the water to clear it of excess soap. When he was ready to be dressed, she again asked his help by holding a piece of clothing for her.

Charles' misconduct was obviously sexually aggressive, but it may also have been a need to do something or a need to "hold onto" something. Louise satisfied his need, which deterred him from acting on his urges. Giving him things to hold onto and helping her in the meantime eliminated this embarrassing situation for Louise.

- Focusing on a desired activity can distract from an undesired one.

- Staying calm and treating a challenge in a quiet way is best.

- Look on unwanted behaviors as opportunities to practice new approaches based on your new knowledge of dementia.

Anecdote—Men and Women Will Always Be Sexual Beings

Jill was a loving woman, determined to keep her husband Mark at home for as long as possible. After a few coaching sessions she said, "I have one problem. When I give him his eye drops he starts to grab at me."

"What does he grab?" I asked.

"He strokes my breasts."

Playfully, I said, "What is wrong with that from your husband? Is it distasteful to you? Does he hurt you?"

"No, it's just that we haven't been sexually active for some time since his diagnosis."

"So, what do you do?" I asked.

"I just usually ignore his behavior and try to hurry up the eye drop installation. But I'm afraid I'll poke his eye one of these times," she said, laughing.

I asked, "If you hugged Mark and he ignored you, what would you feel like?"

"Sad, I guess, like I didn't matter to him, and that I was unattractive to him."

I suggested that he might just need to know she still considered him an attractive man. "Try saying, 'I'm glad you still like my body,' and see what happens," I offered.

She did just that the next week and reported that he withdrew his hands and said, "Yes, you're still beautiful to me."

People with dementia don't stop being male and female; they need affirmation of their sexuality and may want to acknowledge yours. They may just express it in a different way.

Mark was also a restless sleeper and often became disoriented at night. If Jill got out of bed during the night, he would not let her back in, laying crosswise to prevent her from reentering the bed. Sprawled crosswise on the bed he'd say, "You're not sleeping here. I don't know who you are, but you're not getting in my bed." She solved this problem by getting a roll-out couch for the living room!

In the morning Mark was able to recognize her as his wife and all went smoothly thereafter. The repetition of this tired Jill, however, so that in the morning she looked and was tired and often irritable.

Being very tuned into her mood and aware of his need of her, Mark looked concerned. "Are you sick? Are you okay?" Knowing that he felt very dependent on her, Jill decided to again try an appeal to his male ego.

"Well, if you didn't keep me up all night making love, I wouldn't be so tired," she said with hands on her hips and a smile flickering across her face.

He immediately grinned and shrugged. "Well, you're so pretty. I can't help myself."

Fiblets work! Mark was relieved there was a reason for Jill's tiredness and was pleased he was the reason.

- People with dementia need affirmation of their sexual attractiveness.

- Fiblets work!

Anecdote—Respond to the Need to Be Seen as Sexual

This was a second marriage for both George and Linda. They had enjoyed several years of happiness. Both had met at AA meetings and been sober together for ten years. Their relationship had flourished based on trust and mutual support, and they were obviously very much in love. Then George was diagnosed with progressive dementia from Alzheimer's disease. This was devastating news to them, especially Linda, who had been through a bad marriage and felt she had been given a gift in marrying George.

George began becoming disoriented and confused. He would sometimes fail to recognize Linda as his wife, and reverted to living in the past. He thought he still worked as a pastry chef and would say he had to go to work in the mornings. He did not drive, due to his diagnosis, but she let him sit in his beloved car, a 1958 Oldsmobile 98, which usually calmed him. George was a gentle, loving man, very affectionate to Linda.

Linda told me this story on our first coaching visit.

"One night he woke in the night, rolled over toward me and was terrified. He said, 'My wife is coming home. You have to get out of here now! Just take the money on the bureau and leave, now!" he screamed.

Linda had tried to reorient him to her identity. "I am your wife, George. What is the matter?" But this attempt to reorient only made him more fearful that he would be "caught" with another woman: her.

Once before, he had run into the hall of the apartment building yelling for help to "get this woman out of my apartment!" Linda was embarrassed as neighbors called the police, which frightened George so much that he broke their third floor apartment window in an attempt to escape what he perceived as a threat. She was caught in her nightgown, and he was bleeding from his escape attempt.

Linda and I looked at her feelings about this embarrassing misadventure. She wondered if George was cheating on her as he had many years before with his first wife. They had maintained a good sexual relationship throughout the course of the disease, but now she was disinclined to make love to him, wondering if he was faithful. His lack of recognition of her as his wife also made her anxious. Was he just living in a remote past time, or was this a current affair? She wanted to believe he was faithful but didn't know how to respond when he didn't recognize her and demanded she leave. She said, "I feel like a whore."

We decided on an approach. When he told her to leave, I instructed her to say, "Okay, I'm leaving." She would then go to the door of the apartment, open it, close it, wait to the count of twenty-five, open it again, and say, "Hi, George, it's me, Linda. I'm home!"

The next time he had the episode in the night, she did as we planned, with some apprehension about it working. But when she returned to the bedroom door, George cried out, "Oh, I'm so glad you're home, Linda. You can't believe what has been going on here. Strangers have been trying to get in."

George had been in another place in his mind's experience. He was confused and disoriented. Linda simply accommodated his confusion and relieved his fear.

- Look at the behavior as an expression of a feeling, in this case fear, based on past experience.

- Our emotional reaction to a situation can prevent us from finding a workable solution to a seemingly toxic situation.

- Memory loss can be expressed in many and varied behaviors.

Anecdote-Form a Team Approach

Jill was a bright woman who had overcome many challenges in her life. She had learned since George's diagnosis she had to look ahead, planning proactively. When she found people living in the apartment building poking fun at George going "to work" each morning (he was really going to an adult day program), she called a community meeting of all the residents. She hung a poster in the community room inviting everyone to learn about George's disease, Alzheimer's. She called in a representative from the Alzheimer's Association and me to teach the residents about dementia, how to respond to changes in behavior and how they could help George in particular. None of the unhelpful poking fun was mentioned as a reprimand, just what they could do to help Jill and George.

After this meeting handouts were given to all residents that attended and delivered to those that did not. As a result of this informational meeting, the residents' attitude toward George changed radically. They engaged him in conversation as he waited for the van to pick him up, and shared in his joy in working as a chef. With education, others can work in a team effort, greatly aiding the care partner.

Anecdote—Self-soothing or Sexual?

Nancy called me to say "I need some help; it's a sexual thing."

I asked what her husband, John, was doing that was disturbing her.

"He fiddles with himself while we sit together in the living room."

"What do you do? How do you respond?"

"I say 'I don't like when you do that! I am going into the other room until you stop.'"

Asking how he responded, she told me, "He said okay and stopped."

Another time she had said, "It bothers me to see you do that. Will you stop?" Again he willingly stopped holding his genitals. Upon further questioning, Nancy revealed John did not open his pants, nor did he seem to be sexually aroused. He did not pursue sexual activity with Nancy as a result of this activity either.

Pause for thought

How would you handle this same situation if it was your spouse?

_____

_____

_____

_____

_____

Nancy needed to see this behavior in another way. Many people with dementia self soothe. They are fearful and feel lost, and they don't know how to relieve this feeling. Understanding that the purpose of this behavior was probably to relieve boredom, reduce restlessness or to relieve anxiety, Nancy was able to consider John's behavior with different feelings. Instead of getting alarmed, she accepted her husband's need to release feelings or to do something. She acknowledged his restlessness, offering him a snack and her company. Both Nancy and John were able to find comfort in being together once more.

- Sexuality is always an issue whether it gets verbally or behaviorally expressed.

- Each behavior must be taken as an expression of a feeling or a need, but the need may be basic and easily met.

- Respond, don't react, to annoying or puzzling behaviors.

Anecdote—Using Romance to Address a Bathing Challenge

Carlos is a man who speaks several languages, and is a true romantic. He has always been very sexual and still finds his wife safe to be with in his state of dementia. It is important as his disease progresses that he sees her as a safe haven. Lately he has had several episodes a day of wetting himself. This is very embarrassing to him and it makes him agitated. He paces and sometimes leaves the house to pace outdoors. Andrea, his wife, asked the doctor for something to keep him calmer. His physician ordered a tranquilizer, Ativan, for him, but it seemed to make him more restless and agitated. Andrea was afraid of his increasing agitation and wondered why he had suddenly become incontinent.

A person may become incontinent because of the progression of a disease or a medical condition like urinary tract infection. They may have "accidents" because they cannot find the bathroom (spatial disorientation), or get confused about what to do once they get there.

Andrea, who runs a pre-school program in their home, was an easy student to engage in learning approaches. She related many of the behaviors to those of her children who couldn't express their needs easily.

I suggested that incontinence could be due to many things and decided to find out first if Carlos was spatially disoriented and couldn't find his way to the bathroom. The bathroom was down an unlit hallway. Andrea was instructed to put a light in the dark hallway leading to the bathroom and to buy a sign at the hardware store that read GENTLEMEN→→, the arrows leading the way to the bathroom. After these simple interventions we discovered that he hadn't been able to find the bathroom. He now could, and did not have wetting accidents again.

Carlos was also reluctant to shower. Counting on his romantic nature and his physical attraction to her, Andrea dressed in a provocative nightgown and seductively led him down the hallway into the shower. He was very agreeable! Carlos was fully dressed as she led him into the shower. When a person is in wet clothes, the instinct is to take them off. Carlos did as Andrea took off hers. She was mirroring what she wanted him to do. She discovered she enjoyed the closeness as well and it was very soothing to Carlos. She continued to shower him this way for some time.

- Look at challenges as opportunities to keep relationships alive.

- Think creatively outside the Alzheimer's box.

The Couple

They once were a couple
My mom and my dad
Now as they sit and hold hands
She holds the memories he had
He's in the same house he's been in for years
But now as a stranger with confusion and fear
Yet now and again, he will look in her eyes
And remember a trinket from the past that's gone by
And just for that moment, he's back by her side
And her heart fills with warmth, sadness, love and pride

-Judy Paglia

PRESERVING
SELF-ESTEEM

Anecdote—Accommodate Expectations to Cognitive Changes

Jan and Randy was a couple in their late fifties. Jan had just received a diagnosis of early Alzheimer's and expressed sadness about having to give up working at a job she'd had for many years and found great personal satisfaction in. She had been aware for some time that she was having a good deal of difficulty keeping track of phone calls and orders as office manager for the auto parts business. Her ability to concentrate and hold onto a piece of information was gradually worsening. Now, even at home she found herself going into a room and wondering what she was there for, having no memory of the purpose of her trip. All of us do that from time to time, but it was happening to her many times daily.

Randy was unaware of how much trouble Jan was having and continued to give her two pieces of information at a time. "When you go to the living room will you bring back the newspaper, Jan?" Jan would get to the living room and Randy would call out, "While you're there, bring my bottle of water back, too." Jan would stop short, unable to remember what she had come for and unable to bring back two items. Randy would get impatient. "Where's the newspaper? You just brought my water. What is the matter with you anyway? You're losing it." Jan would silently weep, and Randy would feel badly, but the damage had been done. Jan said she felt inadequate and "stupid."

I met with them both and explained how her brain wasn't cooperating with the need to hold onto more than one thought at a time. Concentration and distraction are major challenges for people even in the early stages of Alzheimer's. I explained why Jan wasn't able to cooperate and instructed Randy to give just one request at a time, to make sure he had her attention first, and to avoid adding anything else for Jan to remember or pay attention to until she had completed the first task. Jan was grateful when Randy understood it wasn't something she did deliberately, and Randy learned he had to relate differently to Jan.

Of course, Randy was responding the way he always had, not understanding that Jan's abilities were changing. Working together, they were able to be honest with each other. Jan asked Randy to try to work with her in a different way.

"I'm not stupid, I just have a mind with a mind of its own!" she quipped. Randy agreed to learn and tried very hard to help Jan feel confident. With his added effort to accommodate her memory loss, they began to feel much better about their marital relationship

Changing the way we talk to one another is hard work, particularly difficult for couples. Each partner expects the other to respond in the same way they have for many years. It meant practicing during the coaching session and between sessions to begin to undo old patterns of behavior and adopt new ones. Jan was in the early stage of Alzheimer's and could help Randy by verbally telling him when he slipped back into old habits of communication.

Anecdote—Dementia's Impact on Roles

Jenny and Guy had been together for more than thirty years. Jenny had always been the decision maker, the "capable of anything" type woman, as Guy described her. She had been a skilled company executive and had taught Guy many skills that added to their enjoyment of each other. Guy willingly took care of the cooking, cleaning and food shopping, as Jenny did typically "male" tasks like fixing appliances and repairing household needs.

Then Jenny was diagnosed with Alzheimer's. She began to have trouble multi-tasking, and subsequently had to quit her work. At home she had trouble organizing her day, leaning more and more on Guy to step in and help her. He reported feeling confused by her dependence on him; this was a change in roles.

At first Guy didn't accept the change, denying anything was wrong. He wanted Jenny to maintain the leadership role she had held previously. He would tell her that if she tried harder, she could do whatever the task was. Over time, Guy accepted her inability to complete tasks she had previously done easily. He began to learn how to do what Jenny had always done, and actually began to enjoy the challenge of this new role. Soon he began initiating many of the tasks on his own. Jenny complained of feeling left out of major events and decisions. She felt very hurt and angry toward Guy.

When we talked in our session, Guy talked of his newfound "freedom" with great animation, and his enjoyment in making decisions for them. He seemed unwilling to realize the loss for Jenny. This raised old issues of who was in control, which I found had been an adjustment they felt they had worked out long ago at the beginning of their marriage.

When roles shift, the meaning to each member of the relationship has to be explored to make the transition easier. Feelings may be hurt, resentment can set in and a relationship may suffer irreparably if these problems are not addressed. They are seldom easy transitions and need to be worked out. Jenny and Guy were advised to seek couples counseling to address the changes and their impact on their relationship.

- Challenges are opportunities to keep relationships vital.

- Accommodate, don't take control, to facilitate success.

Anecdote—Reframing to Preserve Self-esteem

Ted was in the cellar when his daughter Anne found him standing in front of the washer and dryer shaking his head. "Can you tell me what is going on here?" he asked. Anne looked; Ted had done the wash over twice and, in addition, had put two cups of detergent in the dryer on top of the dried clothes.

Anne was interested in keeping her father feeling productive and valued. She did not point out his error or his confusion about what he had done. Instead she removed the clothes from the dryer and said, "Let's put these in the wash. Thanks, Dad, for helping. I can use the soap to clean the dryer. It sure needed it!"

"You are welcome," replied Ted. "I thought I'd done something wrong. I'm glad you knew what was going on."

How different that scene could have gone! Anne could have pointed out what errors he had made. She could have complained, "Now look, I have to do the wash all over again! I have enough to do without this mess. What made you put detergent in the dryer, for gosh sake?" This would have embarrassed Ted about an error he couldn't help making. He is confused about the use and operation of objects, and easily distracted. The visual cues of clothes in one machine and clothes in the other mixed him up; dirty clothes are dry when put in the washer and clean clothes are dry when they're done in the dryer.

- Create a situation that enhances the person's value and meaning.

- Avoid criticism of behavior he has no control over.

Anecdote—Handle Social Inappropriateness with Grace

Jayne is a woman who presents well. She is groomed, her face is made up and her hair styled. But when she is out at a restaurant she becomes another person. She is irrational about waiting, demands attention from the wait staff and embarrasses her husband Ed. Because she cannot organize to cook anymore and becomes irate if anyone else tries to cook in her kitchen, eating at restaurants seems to be a solution. Ed decided to ease his embarrassment some by clueing the wait staff about his wife's dementia.

He made up a bogus business card that says

MY WIFE HAS ALZHEIMER'S.

PLEASE BE PATIENT.

When he gives the server this card, Jayne occasionally asks, "What are you giving her?"

He responds, "My business card. We need to give out our business card to everyone we meet, Jayne." If Jayne wants to see it, he produces another real business card and she is satisfied.

This is a good way to prepare strangers for some inappropriate behavior that might surface without embarrassing (or infuriating) the person with dementia and the care partner. Sometimes wait staff will react to you taking charge, perhaps ordering for your family member or cutting her meat. Prepare them with a card and often they will be more understanding.

- Whenever possible, avoid embarrassment for you and your family member with dementia.

- Think ahead to help preserve dignity for them.

- You can help educate public service people about how to work with a person with dementia.

Anecdote—Using Responses that Support Self-esteem

I had been working with Norman and his family for a time, coaching them in responding to his decline in skills more effectively. Ellen and Norman had enjoyed a happy marriage for fifty years. I was visiting with Ellen and their daughter, Susan, in their kitchen. Norm was upstairs where he spent a good portion of the day "sweeping up" rooms contentedly. This activity was good for Norman, who had high energy level. We discovered that working off energy even in seemingly useless activity curbed his need to "go walking." Norman and Ellen lived in a busy part of town. To get to any store, they needed to cross two heavily trafficked streets. We weren't sure Norman was safe to do this, in spite of his familiarity with the neighborhood, so his going walking was a concern for all of us.

Norman soon joined us in the kitchen, appropriately dressed in slacks, a sport shirt, shoes and socks. There was one mistake; he had put his boxer shorts over his trousers. His sequencing skills waning, he had probably dressed and found he had one piece of clothing left over: his boxer shorts. He might have hidden them or, like he did this time, simply put them on over his outer clothes.

Pause for thought

How would you respond to Norman's dress to avoid embarrassing him?

_____
_____
_____
_____
_____

Ellen could have said, "Norman, look at you. You put your underwear on wrong. They go under your trousers!" This would have embarrassed him, pointing out his difficulty sequencing.

Instead she responded, "You look nice, Norman. You always like something soft next to your skin. Perhaps you should try putting those shorts on under your trousers."

Norman looked down at his shorts. "You know, I looked in the mirror and said, 'Something is wrong with this picture,' but couldn't figure it out. Thanks, I'll go change." He proceeded to go upstairs chuckling to himself, and came down with the boxer shorts under his trousers. He had maintained his sense of self-assurance and was spared embarrassment. Ellen had given Norman credit for effort without criticizing him. Instead she appealed to his sense of physical comfort, information she had based on their long history together.

- Strengthen remaining skills by simplifying the task.

- Make the person feel good about himself in relationship to others as often as possible.

- Always treat him with dignity, preserving his sense of self-efficacy.

- Laying out clothing in a pile with the first thing to go on at the top, etc., can help a person dress successfully.

Anecdote—Avoid Embarrassment; Enter Their World

It was my first visit with Michael, a man of seventy-four. As I entered the home, he greeted me with, "Come see what she did in the night while I was sleeping!" I had to smile when he opened the refrigerator and freezer doors. There on each shelf were crystal goblets Anna had lined up.

"I hope you thanked her for chilling the glasses," I offered.

"Is that what I was supposed to do? I blew a gasket at her. I guess I need help. I don't understand why she is doing such crazy things."

"It makes sense to her at the time. She is in a different world. I'll teach you about her world, okay?"

We had just finished talking in the kitchen about his concerns when his wife Anna appeared from the living room where she had been watching a cooking show with her son. She approached me, smiled and said, "You've shortened your hair since I saw you last. And you wear glasses now. When did that happen?"

I responded, "Well, we are getting older, Anna. I have to wear glasses."

We continued this social conversation for a few minutes more until Mike escorted me to my car. "Do you know Anna from somewhere?" he asked.

"No," I replied.

"Then why did you pretend to?"

"To keep her from embarrassment; what good would have come from my telling her I'd never met her before? Besides, having left her with a good feeling about my visit will allow me to come back into a friendly household!"

- Do not refute their sense of reality; enter it.

- Avoid embarrassing a person; do not point out errors.

Nursing Home Halls

They wander the halls
Their eyes far away
They don't know who you are
Or what day is today
In a world of their own
Right in front of your eyes
Every now and then
Stopping in to say "hi."

-Judy Paglia, a daughter

Challenge #10:
MOVING ON: LIVING TO A NEW HOME

The year was 1992. My mom woke to join me for breakfast as usual. Munching on her English muffin she casually remarked, "Well it is time I moved on."

I laughed. "Oh sure, at eighty-five years old you are moving on? Where are you moving to, Mom?"

"I'm going to what is called a life care community in Cheshire, Connecticut, just south of Hartford. I already have been accepted."

"Why are you leaving? You've always been happy here," I asked, concerned.

"I don't feel I want to stay now that you have a new husband (I'd just been married after being widowed fifteen years), not like my mother did. That was hard on your daddy and me. Besides, I'm not feeling safe being alone all day. With my vision going I'm burning my hands cooking in the toaster oven, and I'm finding it harder to take care of myself."

And she did move, in spite of our offering in-home care and contrary to what both my new husband and I wanted. I would miss our daily breakfasts together. Both he and I were enjoying having her living with us, and in addition, Hartford was a three-hour round trip by car!

My mother did not have dementia. It is rare when an elder decides independently to live somewhere else. Usually the people who care for an elder must make that decision, and it is usually a difficult transition for all concerned. (Even though my mom had decided this move herself, I still grieved the loss and felt badly she hadn't felt safe enough in our home.)

So, when is the right time? How do you know? How can we make it happen with the least strain on everyone? These are all good questions.

When the elder has dementia, it is wise not to discuss the move or plan it with him. Remember the reason for not planning with a person with memory loss: it will leave him with anxiety; and, as he is unable to understand the meaning of a move, you would be creating an uncomfortable anticipation for him. There would probably be change in behavior as a result of the fear of the unknown. You want to avoid that discomfort for them. So, prepare the move, and avoid sharing plans with him.

When do you know that a move may be the right thing to do? There are clues that living at home is not the best place.

- When the person is restless at home and unable to structure meaningful activity, and this leads to pacing, retreating, wandering or experiencing irritability or agitation.

- When she shadows (follows) her care partner, a sign of anxiety about being on her own.

- When he is seemingly more content in a structured environment like a day program than at home.

- When care is so burdensome that you get sick, can't sleep, are hyper-vigilant or chronically impatient with her.

- When there is a persistent paranoia or a psychotic condition that warrants supervision and/or medical attention you cannot provide.

Plan ahead and research alternative places for him to live before a crisis occurs. This takes some planning, asking questions and assessing the finances needed to secure a suitable place.

Would an assisted living environment be suitable? This is a residence, generally privately paid for, that offers hands-on help with everyday hygiene tasks such as bathing and dressing, and medication reminders. Such residences offer an activity program geared to entertain, enlighten or provide for using previously learned skills like knitting, painting, dancing, exercise, etc. This is planned by the activities director.

Some assisted living residences offer dementia care in a secure unit within the residence. The ratio of resident-to-staff is much smaller to allow for individualized attention. Activities that are fail-free offer opportunity for residents to be successful. "It is like she is a large fish in a small pond, rather than a small fish in a large pond," one person described her mom. "Once she moved out of the larger residence to the dementia unit she seemed much happier."

Nursing homes are another option; usually this choice is made when the person is unable to care for herself adequately and needs nursing care. A memory impaired person needs a very structured setting to thrive; a dementia unit in a nursing home provides this and the nursing care needed.

You can ask a person from each type of living arrangement to evaluate your family member for what level of care is needed. Facilities want to provide the care that will enhance life for the elder.

What to look for in an alternative living environment:

• An Alzheimer's friendly environment

- Soothing colors, sometimes color-contrasted to guide residents to designated rooms

- Stimulation without disturbance from too much stimulation

- Friendly, attentive staff

- Staff trained in the habilitation approach to care

- Gives good eye contact

- Speaks slowly, clearly and reassuringly

- Does not reprimand a resident

- Proactively approaches a resident expressing a need for attention

- Low volume noise as the rule

- A meaningful activity program; fail-free activities

- Smells are pleasant or minimally offensive (and then, not usual)

- Clean environment, uncluttered, with good unobstructed pathways for walking

- Soft lighting, no fluorescent lighting

- Floors are not shiny, which confuses residents

Making the Move: Prepare Ahead

- Do not ask him if he wants to move.

- Do not threaten with a move when he is ill behaved.

- Do not talk about the move in advance.o This just makes the person anxious. He has no memory of what is to happen, but is left with an uneasy feeling something bad is about to happen. This may lead to perseveration.

Prepare Yourself:

Reframe this difficult move for yourself: the new living space should be:

- a more suitable home

- safer

- enhancing life for her

Remember:

- I'm not giving up on him.

- I'm not "putting him away."

- It is not that I've failed him.

What to Expect after the Move

There will be an adjustment period for you after moving your relative to a new home. No matter how you've reasoned in your head and your heart that it is a good choice, it will be challenge for you to come to peace with your decision. Expect this and work through the feelings! This move is one of the most difficult times emotionally for us all. We question our wisdom and our commitment to our family member, and we second guess our decision.

The staff may suggest that you don't visit for a time (a few days to a week or more) to ease the change in living space, routine and care partners. This is in your best interest, too. She may want to leave with you each time you visit, even if she is demonstrating comfort there, and it will add to your inner emotional turmoil. Your presence reminds her of a previous familiar time and place. However, once you leave, she may indeed settle into the routine there without fuss.

You can help the transition for yourself and her by establishing a team approach. Tell the staff you want to work with them, to be part of the treatment team. This is proactive and assuring for the staff. It is good to point out positive things that the staff does and to thank them for their good work. We all need affirmation, and the people that work in a memory impairment unit choose to do that kind of work. They deserve our appreciation. Compliment good care liberally. If you have a complaint, explore with the staff the reasons behind your concern. Avoid blaming. It just sets up barriers and will not be helpful to sustaining the team.

Your family member needs time to adjust as well. When I brought my mother-in-law to her room in the nursing home, she looked at her things and cried, "I can't do this. Don't make me do this!"

I wrapped my arms around her as she cried. "Sometimes things don't turn out the way we'd like," I offered.

She insisted, "I'm taking a train home to Maine. I'm not staying here."

She was obviously frightened and showed her fear the way she always had: in angry threats. I said little more, simply held her. She was in an emotional place I couldn't go. She needed to make the adjustment with staff help.

Within two days she was calm and engaging in activities on the unit. Staff members were able to make her welcome because of a short bio-sketch paper. I recommend this to families when there is a change of caregivers, whether the elder is entering a day program or receiving in-home help. It gives information that can help the new caregivers "join" with the elder.

I had written a one-page description of Betty's family of origin, the family she raised with her husband, her interests, skills she had, like pastel painting, and her likes and dislikes in food. I described typical behaviors and how to respond to them most effectively. I included a photo of a smiling, healthier Betty. The report was placed inside a three-hole plastic sleeve so that it could be inserted inside the front cover of her chart.

The staff said it was very helpful; it told them she'd "do anything" for chocolate or for her son, Curt. It told them when she resisted treatment to say that Curt asked them to do this for her and would be angry if they didn't comply. The report also told them she hates licorice, broccoli and milk. I wrote this to help them help my mother-in-law successfully.

What Do I Do Now that the Caregiving Is Over?

First, understand that your role as care partner is not over. Your frequent contact with the staff at the new home is important to ensure good continuity of care. Your care partnering now is one of an advocate, a liaison between your family member and the staff. Different staff come on every eight hours, and each staff member will need your teaming with them to make care go more smoothly.

Sometimes you will find things you don't like, ways you found worked for you that the staff is not doing in the same way. It is good to make suggestions that will be helpful but to also understand that your family member will respond to staff differently from the way they did to you. But, you can be a good teacher of approaches that did work for you.

For example, I learned that my mother in law was almost combative when being dressed. She would shove against the aide and fret, wringing her hands. I often found her dressed in clothes that were not hers in spite of her closet being full of her own wardrobe. This not only concerned me that she was combative but also annoyed me she wasn't wearing her own clothes. I wondered if she was being given choices about what to wear. And if she was being dressed in another person's clothes, was that what was driving her reaction to retaliate? I told the staff that she only wore pastels and that she needed to have choices but no more than two. I was doing her laundry so I hung outfits that went together that I knew would please her taste. I made a sign on her closet door:

PLEASE DRESS BETTY IN HER OWN CLOTHES.
SLIPS, PANTIES AND SOCKS ARE IN THE PLASTIC BASKET.

I provided a plastic container they could put her slips, panties and socks in to make them easier to find. Staff can be very busy in the mornings helping all the residents dress. They may have just been taking the easiest, most available clothing they saw. Soon I noticed that Betty was being dressed in her own clothes, and I learned that her irritability around dressing had lessened considerably. She felt in control again choosing what to wear, something she is still capable of doing.

How Can I Have a Good Visit in My Mom's New Home?

There's a little story to I must tell you to answer this question. When visiting my mother years ago in a nursing home, although she did not have dementia, she was in a slower-paced world. I was just starting this coaching business, and being busy educating professionals about the value of my service, I would run in to spend a short time with my mother a few times a day, whenever there was a break in my schedule. One morning, as I rushed into the nursing home, a resident stuck out her leg, nearly tripping me. She said, "You aren't any earthly good as a visitor! You rush in, rush out, looking like you're on a treadmill. Why do you visit at all?" Her remarks first shocked and annoyed me, but then they made me stop and think. Was my visit good at all for mom? I asked my mother, who has always been very honest with me about her thoughts.

"Sometimes I wish you hadn't come. Sometimes you're not really present at all. You're already thinking of somewhere else," she replied.

I left slowly, thinking about her remarks. When at home, I sat down and wrote the following Good Visit to help me visit my mother well. Many families have told me it has been very helpful for them. I hope it is helpful for you as well.

The Good Visit

So you visit with someone who has Alzheimer's disease or dementia from another memory disorder! You live in two different realities: theirs and yours. Yours, no doubt, is faster paced, rapidly switching from one activity to another, and noisy. Theirs is slowed, quieter, based in the remote past, which is a predictable place in its familiarity of people and routines. Can these two realities meet for long enough to make a good visit?

Yes. You must meet them in their reality. You are the one who must accommodate them. A person with dementia cannot sustain staying in the present; it is too difficult and confusing. They will often retreat in their mind to a time and place they understood, a place in which they felt safe and loved. Go there with them and you will have a better than good visit.

Here are some helpful tips to get you on your way.

Plan a time limit on your visit, one that you can handle with grace.

Slow down your pace and your mind before entering their space.

Identify yourself each time. If they don't know who you are, introduce yourself by your first name, "Hi, Mom, Brad your son is here to spend some time with you." *It may take a full minute* for her to orient to your being there and who you are.

State what day and time it is. Then, *wait* for them to absorb this information.

Stimulate conversation with a sentence and *wait.* Sometimes it takes a full minute or longer for the brain to accept the message, make some sense of it and formulate a response. So, wait the minute.

Don't jump from subject to subject.

Plan a task or activity you can accomplish while you're there: a short walk with *easy, slow* talk (you'll probably carry most of the conversation), reading a story or listening to music together, a manicure, a foot soak, mouth care or hair brushing (with the usually comforting human touch).

Communicate positive feelings through quiet hand holding, kisses (when appropriate), a light back rub, a hand resting on her back or forearm. *Always approach from the front before touching them so they don't startle.*

Talk slowly and deliberately. Repeat parts as necessary to be clear.

Avoid arguing with their perceptions of things. Sometimes saying nothing works best. (P.S. You *always* lose an argument with a confused person!)

Enjoy being in their world. *Play* in it with them.

Do not reality orient or correct their memories or perceptions of things.

Avoid questioning and quizzing (these are actually unkind). Give information instead.

When asking them to choose something, *offer only two choices,* either of which is acceptable. More than that is too much for the brain to deal with now. E.g., "Do you want to walk with me now, or share these cookies first?"

Try breathing and moving deliberately. It will be beneficial for you and them (mood is contagious).

Be aware that *your presence alone* may be enough to bring peace and comfort to their confusing and often frightening world.

Practicing these can be meditative. You'll learn great patience and have a sense of peacefulness. That is good for you! You will also enjoy yourself as you sense the joy you bring to them.

Now, wasn't that a good visit?

Getting on with Your Life

Sometimes it is hard to see yourself apart from the hands-on caregiving role. It is important that you do, however. You must get on with your life and find meaning outside of caregiving. There is a grieving process for this loss. You've identified yourself with caring for someone you love, and now you must care for you! How do you do that?

Explore new ways to bring meaning to your life. Renew old interests; renew contact with family members you didn't make time to connect with. You must also forgive hurts: yours. The family that didn't come forth to help is still there. Reconnect. They did what they had to do and you did what you had to do. Harboring resentment only hurts you and prevents reestablishing family ties.

At a talk on caregiving a few years ago I met a woman who had taken care of her aunt and her mother for several years. She had been a real estate broker before deciding to be a full time caregiver. She said that once the caregiving was over, she found no interest in returning to selling real estate. "I had found a new career: that of a caregiver. I found such satisfaction in my new role; it was so much more meaningful to me than selling properties. I decided then to go into elder health care. I volunteer. I take care of myself by running each morning and having a devotional time, which centers me. Then I go to the local council on aging to volunteer my time. It is the way I find fulfillment now."

Grieving is anticipatory and real. You must allow yourself to grieve the loss of a partner, your care recipient, your job as caregiver. You should anticipate this throughout the illness of dementia. You grieve with each downward slip in ability and behavior. You grieve the loss of the person who was and the reality of the person he has become.

Grieving takes on many stages. When my mother died after a long illness, I sensed no sadness, just relief in the end to her suffering. Six months after her death, I began having a choking feeling in my throat and didn't want to eat. I lost twenty-five pounds. I found myself tearful at every red light while driving to and from client appointments.

I soon joined a bereavement group offered by the hospice that had served my mother in her last year of life. In the group, I also found myself grieving for my first husband who had died some thirty years before. This puzzled me. The leader said, "You never grieved him. You are doing it now. Grief is accumulative. So when you lost your mother, you relived losing your husband." I had been thirty-two at his death, with two small children to tend to, so I swallowed my grief and went on as best I could. Now that I look back, some of my new strange behaviors in the days following his death were unhelpful expressions of grief. So, grieve your losses. Allow yourself to adjust to being without your role, your relative.

Care partnering changes you. You stretch yourself, sometimes seemingly beyond your limits, to give to someone special to you. In the meantime you are transformed. Like one support group attendee said, "I learned I had the capacity for compassion; what a lovely thing to learn about myself."

What have you learned about yourself since assuming the care of someone with a memory disorder? Have you, like he, discovered traits of yours you never were aware of? Have you developed new behaviors outside of the care partnering experience?

Much of what we learn while care partnering is transferable to other relationships; we find we have increased empathy, do more listening than talking and observe body language more closely. This skill teaches us a way to read another's feelings, so we can respond better.

I have a poster in my office that reads:

What You Get by Achieving Your Goals Is Not as Important as What You Become by Achieving Your Goals

-Zig Ziglar

You've reached your goal. What have you become?

Postscript

Writing this guide for you has been a pleasure. As I write, I learn again what has worked. Reading it over brings to mind the many hundreds of willing families who didn't accept that a diagnosis of Alzheimer's means doom. They knew that knowledge is power—and facing a disease like Alzheimer's does make one feel powerless. They launched out to learn all that was available in books, on the Internet, in support groups and through a coach and their local or state Alzheimer's Association.

I am reminded of a class I taught as part of a graduate course called Counseling Adolescents. The class was entitled "What's in a Label," reminding the professionals in the course to avoid putting their adolescent clients into the confines of a label. I would remind you to think outside the box labeled Alzheimer's and look at your family member as uniquely expressing himself through the disease. Do not expect the worst; hope for the best. You can make it happen daily.

In January 2008, Alzheimer's Coaching Services enters its ninth year serving families. I feel blessed to be doing work that can combine all the skills I've developed as a medical nurse, a family therapist, a mental health clinician, an educator, a parent, a wife, a member of a family (or two) and a trainer and support group facilitator. I am passing on my learning to you and to the coaches on my staff. In my sixth decade of life, I want to be sure my work coaching families is carried on well. I'm planning on being here for another three decades, at least, learning more from families like you.

In the beginning of the book, I said this was not an all-inclusive study of dementia. I confined it to what I know best: behavior. After all, it is what people do that is a delight or a challenge to us. I could continue writing this book for a lifetime. Each time I meet with a family, I learn something new I want to pass on to you. Perhaps there will have to be a second edition some day.

I would be pleased to hear from you via e-mail at Alzheimer-coaching@juno.com. I value your opinion on what was helpful and what else might have been included in the book. Also, check my web-site at www.alzheimercoachingservice.com.

Some "Cheat Sheets" to Help You on Your Way:

Tips for Relating to People with Memory Loss

How a person with memory loss thinks differently:

- Thinking is slower so understanding takes longer.

- Remembering is hard at first, then perhaps impossible.

- What he remembers may be different from what you remember.

- Understanding explanations is hard.

- Time and sequence of events may be distorted.

- Social appropriateness may be lacking.

- Organizing and doing tasks in the right order is more difficult.

- It is harder to pay attention and concentrate on something.

- Memory for recent events is lost before memory for events of the distant past.

How you can help by relating differently:

- Say her name first, and then start speaking to her.

- Turn off background noises when having a conversation.

- Maintain his attention; use eye contact.

- Speak slowly and simply; avoid complex concepts.

- Stay on one subject; avoid switching the subject mid-sentence.

- Avoid long explanations, e.g., why she must do something.

- Avoid questions asking what, who, when, and especially why. Use questions that can be answered yes or no.

- Repeat information as necessary.

- Apologize if you've expected too much or been rushed.

- Encourage participation in family life; this gives life meaning.

- Go slowly when doing something and do it together if you can.

- Do not correct him if he is wrong; do not argue with what he thinks is true.

- Treat her with respect. She needs to know that she is important to you.

- Understand that his behavior is his way of staying in touch with what is going on to feel in control of his life.

More Practical Tips for Working with People with Dementia

These tips are based on principles of dementia care born out of an understanding of brain dysfunction and resulting behaviors.

- Slow down your speech and action to match hers.

- Stay on one subject at a time; maintain eye contact.

- Simplify everything; success becomes more achievable.

- Satisfy the immediate emotional need (reassurance, recognition).

- Fiblets are used to satisfy the immediate emotional need.

- Avoid use of logic and reason; it is too hard to process.

- Avoid explaining why something must be done; just state the task.

- Focus on one activity to distract from an undesired one.

- Use memory loss to defuse potential or real explosive situations.

- Point out the positive behaviors and avoid criticizing negative ones.

- Mood is contagious; exhibit the mood you want him to be in.

- Get into the reality of the moment and stay there with her.

- Address sexuality expressed behaviorally or verbally; it is often an expression of feeling unattractive or disempowered.

- Mirroring a behavior jump-starts the mind's memory for doing it.

- Inform rather than reorient; avoid quizzing.

- Accommodate, not control, to facilitate success.

- Give choices as often as possible; limit him to two. It empowers.

- "Home" is a place of emotional safety, not necessarily the actual home. Offer emotional safety to make her feel at home within.

- Wandering is often a search for someone or some place familiar.

- Staying active prevents many unwanted symptoms such as pacing, wandering, rummaging, irritability and restlessness.

Structuring Time through Activities

Presenting Activities for Person(s) with Dementia

- Modify according to the person's needs, abilities and limitations.

- Base the activity on the familiar.

- Make it simple with few steps.

- Allow for passive participation (perhaps watching you do it).

- Encourage any opportunity to be helpful (people need to be needed).

- Make it an opportunity for socialization (this may be the main goal).

- Choose a concrete activity.

- Make it fun, enjoyable and success-oriented.

How to Start

- Initiate activity yourself; ask them to join you.

- Give visual demonstration and perhaps examples.

- Ask for their assistance (again, people need to feel needed).

- You may have to use a step-by-step method (called "chunking").

- Always treat the person as an adult.

Achieving Success

- Be sensitive to the person's needs and interests.

- Be flexible and creative.

- Be an initiator (remember that they cannot initiate activity easily).

- Never criticize; praise generously.

- Make room for communication of feelings.

- Use eye-to-eye contact, touch and body language to focus them.

- Keep a sense of humor!

Types of Activities

- Cognitive: crossword puzzles, fill in the blank, complete a song, proverb or saying, matching games, guessing games

- Physical activities: exercise, games with balls, bean bags, walking

- Sensory stimulation: Use any activity that stimulates sight, sound, feel (tactile), taste or smell, i.e., baking, candles, soft stuffed animals. *** The sensory activities are some of the few that can be continued late in the disease and bring much pleasure to the person.

- Hand/eye coordination: Stacking, sorting (clothes, socks, silverware, coins, matching socks) and moving (building blocks and Legos are great to do with small children; it brings the adult into a helping role easily).

Passive Activities

- Pictures (catalogues, books of interest, pets, making a scrapbook)

- Reading (the Bible, Chicken Soup for the Soul, prayer books, simple poetry)

- Music (sing-along, hymns, era songs)

- Jokes and riddles

- Specific TV shows (with accompanying discussion of themes)—Do not use TV as a babysitter!

Games & Puzzles: cards, Bingo, checkers, dominoes, large piece puzzles (no more than 350 pieces is best; later, when abilities decline, 100 pieces may be enough), matching cards, Hangman, Trivia

Crafts: painting, coloring, cutting, special projects suited to interest/ability

Household activities: food preparation, cooking, washing dishes or clothes, bedmaking, gardening, watering, sweeping, dusting, dry mopping, folding laundry, stacking, i.e., wood, bricks, boxes, etc.

Musical Activities: singing, dancing, playing instruments, listening to others performing

Any activity stimulates brain connections, so any creative way you can engage them in life is worth trying. If at first they don't seem interested, don't give up. Try another time or change the activity or do it for a shorter time period.

This list was derived from the Atlanta Area Chapter of the Alzheimer's Association, 3120 Raymond Drive, Atlanta, GA 30340

Other Resources to Help You

- The Alzheimer's Association: each state has its own association chapter. In Massachusetts it is www.alzmass.org. Look up your local Association on the Internet.

- www.alz.org, the national website for information about Alzheimer's disease including resources, research participation opportunities, partnerships, Alzheimer's friendly professionals; legal, medical, financial, etc

- The Safe Return Program: a program to return people to their care partners. Call the National Alzheimer's Association for an application 1-888-572-8566. There is presently a $40 fee for the bracelet and $5 extra for a care partner bracelet.

- Support groups for caregivers; ask your state aging service agency and local council on aging. There are specialized groups for the challenges of various diseases and disorders that cause dementia. The Alzheimer's Association in your area should also have a list of support groups in your area. Check their website.

- www.theazheimersstore.com, which carries unique products to ease the care of someone with a cognitive disorder

- Adult day programs: structured activities for filling the day with meaningful social contact and creativity in a failure-free atmosphere

- www.caremanager.org: a list of Professional Geriatric Care Managers (PGCM), elder care specialists who assist older adults and their families to develop and implement a comprehensive plan to optimize safety, independence and comfort for the elder

- www.gcmnewengland.com, the New England website for information in geriatric care managers

- www.caregiverscoach.com, an online chat room to share experiences with other caregivers, especially good if you are unable to find a way to get to a support group

Fine Books I've Enjoyed Learning from

Alzheimer's: A Caregiver's Guide and Sourcebook by Howard Gruetzner; John Wiley and Sons, Inc. New York, 1992.

Alzheimer's Early Stages: First Steps in Caring and Treatment by Daniel Kuhn, MSW; Hunter House Publishers, Inc., California 1998.

Care for People with Alzheimer's Disease: A Training Manual for Community Care Providers by Joanne Koenig-Coste, M.Ed; published by the Alzheimer's Association of Eastern Massachusetts, Cambridge, Massachusetts, 1998.

Care That Works: A Relationship Approach to Persons with Dementia by Jitka M. Zgola; Johns Hopkins University Press, Baltimore and London, 1999.

Doing Things: A Guide to Programming Activities for Persons with Alzheimer's Disease and Related Disorders by Jitka M. Zgola; John Hopkins University Press, Baltimore and London, 1987.

Counseling the Alzheimer's Caregiver by Mary S. Mittelman, Cynthia Epstein and Alicia Pierzchala; AMA Press 2003. (This is a good read for professionals.)

The 36-Hour Day by Nancy L. Mace and Peter V. Rabins; Johns Hopkins University Press, 1999 (called the Alzheimer's bible).

Learning to Speak Alzheimers by Joanne Koenig Coste; Houghton Mifflin Company, Boston and New York, 2003 (a personal story of care partnering with numerous resources and care tips.)

Understanding Difficult Behaviors: Some Practical Suggestions for Coping with Alzheimer's Disease and Related Illnesses by Anne Robinson; Beth Spenser and Laurie White, editors; published by the Geriatric Education Center of Michigan, 1988.

Alzheimer's—Finding the Words: A Communication Guide for Those Who Care by Harriet Hodgson; John Wiley & Sons, Inc., New York, 1995.

Rethinking Alzheimer's Care by Sam Fazio, Dorothy Seman, and Jane Stansell; Health Professions Press, Baltimore, London, Winnipeg and Sidney.

The Alzheimer's Caregiver by Harriet Hodgson, Chronimed Publishing, Minneapolis, Minnesota, 1998.

The Forgetting; Alzheimer's Portrait of an Epidemic by David Shenk; Anchor Books, New York, New York, 2001.

Voices of Alzheimer's by Betsy Peterson; Da Capo Lifelong Press, Cambridge, Massachusetts, 2004 (thoughts from those with memory loss and those who care about them).

The New Peoplemaking by Virginia Satir; Science and Behavior Books, Inc., Mountain View, California, 1988 (an older humorous book about family relationships and styles of relating).

The Magic Tape Recorder: A Story about Growing Up and Growing Down by Joyce Simard, MSW; Joyce Simard Publishing and Czech Alzheimer's Society, Land O Lakes, Florida and the Czech Republic, 2007 (a wonderful colorful, washable book to help children understand memory loss).

The Everything Alzheimer's Book: Reliable Accessible Information for Patients and Their Families by Carolyn Dean, M.D., N.D.; Adams Media, a F+W Publications, Inc., Avon, Massachusetts 2004 (includes information about diet, nutrients and the value of exercise and prevention.)

Testimonials

It was in talking and working with Beverly that I found confidence and hope. She helped me with some of the most difficult times and decisions I had to face during my husband's fight with Alzheimer's.

--ALMA IN CANTON

I always looked forward to Beverly's visit. She would tell me ways to make tasks like showering my husband work. In my eyes she was my guardian angel.

--FLORENCE IN ASSONET

I learned how to touch my husband's emotions.

--ANN FROM REHOBOTH

Beverly is a brilliant coach with a gentle heart. She taught me how to live in my husband's world. He is a child in a man's body needing love and my telling him how great he is...because he is.

--CHARLOTTE

I learned how to say things in a different way. What a difference.

--CAROL, A DAUGHTER

Printed in the United States
104210LV00002B/76-99/P

9 781599 320632